100 Data Interpretation Questions for the MRCP

100 Data Interpretation Questions for the MRCP

Michael D. Flynn MB MRCP
Research Fellow, King's College Hospital, London

Richard F. U. Ashford MA MB MRCP FRCR
Consultant Radiotherapist and Oncologist, Mount Vernon Hospital,
Middlesex, and The Cromwell Hospital, London

Patrick J. W. Venables MD MRCP
Senior Lecturer in Rheumatology,
Charing Cross Hospital, London

SECOND EDITION

Churchill Livingstone ▓
EDINBURGH LONDON MELBOURNE AND NEW YORK 1987

CHURCHILL LIVINGSTONE
Medical Division of Longman Group UK Limited

Distributed in the United States of America by
Churchill Livingstone Inc., 1560 Broadway, New York,
N.Y. 10036, and by associated companies, branches
and representatives throughout the world.

First Edition 1979
  Reprinted 1981
Second Edition 1987

ISBN 0-443-03779-5

British Library Cataloguing in Publication Data
Ashford, Richard
    100 data interpretation questions for
    the MRCP.—2nd ed.
    1. Diagnosis—Problems, exercises, etc.
    I. Title II. Flynn, Michael D.
    III. Venables, Patrick
    616.07'5'076   RC71.3

Library of Congress Cataloging in Publication Data
Flynn, Michael D.
    100 data interpretation questions for the MRCP.
    Rev. ed. of: 100 data interpretation questions for
    the MRCP/ by Richard Ashford and Patrick Venables.
    1st ed. 1979.
    1. Diagnosis, Laboratory—Examinations, questions,
    etc. I. Ashford, Richard. II. Venables, Patrick. III.
    Ashford, Richard. 100 data interpretation questions for
    the MRCP. IV. Title. V. Title: One hundred data
    interpretation questions for the MRCP. [DNLM: 1.
    Diagnosis, Laboratory—examination questions. QY
    18 F648z] RB37.F59 1987   616.07'5'076
    87-761

Produced by Longman Publisher Pte Ltd
Printed in Singapore

Preface to the Second Edition

The main aim of this book is to enable the reader to assess his or her ability to make reasonable deductions from laboratory data; we also aim to entertain.

For the Second Edition the questions have all been carefully revised and many new questions have been added, to reflect changes in medical practice since publication of the First Edition. The questions cover a wide variety of clinical conditions and are arranged in a layout similar to the MRCP part II, with ten papers each consisting of two ECGs and eight other questions covering endocrinology, chemical pathology, haematology, lung function and cardiac catheter data. Most of the questions and all of the ECGs are based on patients seen by us or our colleagues, although some of the information has been modified to avoid it being misleading and to take account of variation between reference ranges produced by different hospitals.

In each case an answer is provided and a differential diagnosis discussed. The book is not intended to be a text book, but to provoke thought, expose hidden areas of ignorance and act as an aid to data interpretation

The veracity of every question has been carefully checked by independent experts and we are grateful to Dr J. Silva, Dr R. Sutton and Dr D. Samson for checking data used in the First Edition, and to Dr P. Drury, Dr T. Cundy and Dr M. Hammer for checking the revised and new data for the Second Edition.

London 1987

M.D.F.
R.F.U.A.
P.J.W.V.

CONTENTS

Tables of reference ranges

Plasma or serum

	Units
Alanine transminase (ALT)	$\leq$ 35 iu/l
Albumin	35–45 g/l
Alkaline phosphatase	20–100 iu/l
Aspartate transaminase (AST)	$\leq$ 30 iu/l
Bicarbonate	22–28 mmol/l
Bilirubin	5–17 µmol/l
Calcium	2.2–2.6 mmol/l
Chloride	95–105 mmol/l
Cholesterol	3.4–6.5 mmol/l
Creatinine	42–130 µmol/l
Creatinine Phosphokinase (CPK)	$\leq$ 195 iu/l
Iron	11–32 µmol/l
Iron binding capacity (TIBC)	45–78 µmol/l
Magnesium	0.65–0.96 mmol/l
Osmolality	285–295 mosm/kg
Phosphate	0.8–1.4 mmol/l
Potassium	3.5–5.0 mmol/l
Protein (total)	58–80 g/l
Sodium	135–145 mmol/l
Urea	2.5–6.5 mmol/l
γ-Glutamyl transpeptidase	$\leq$ 50 iu/l
Immunoglobulins	
IgA	0.5–3.2 g/l
IgG	5.5–14.5 g/l
IgM	0.5–3.1 g/l

Hormones

Cortisol	
9 am	180–700 nmol/l
midnight	up to 180 nmol/l
Follicle stimulating hormone (FSH)	
Male	1–7 iu/l
Post menopausal	28–130 iu/l

Luteinising hormone (LH)
  Male   2.5–10 iu/l
  Post menopausal   29–120 iu/l
Prolactin   < 600 mu/l
Testosterone (male)   13–30 nmol/l
Thyroxine   60–160 nmol/l
Thyroid stimulating hormone (TSH)   0.4–5.0 mu/l
Free T4   8.8–23 pmol/l

Values for other investigations are given in the answers to the relevant questions.

Haematological

Haemoglobin (Hb)
  male   13.5–18.0 g/dl
  female   11.5–16.5 g/dl
Red blood cell count
  male $4.5–6.5 \times 10^{12}/l$
  female $3.9–5.6 \times 10^{12}/l$
Packed cell volume
  male   0.4–0.54%
  female   0.35–0.47%
Mean corpuscular haemoglobin (MCH)   27–32 pg
Mean corpuscular haemoglobin
concentration (MCHC)   30–36 g/dl
Mean corpuscular volume (MCV)   76–98 fl
Platelets $150–400 \times 10^{9}/l$
Reticulocytes   0.2–2.0%
White blood cells (WBC) $4.0–11.0 \times 10^{9}/l$
Neutrophils $2.0–7.5 \times 10^{9}/l$
Lymphocytes $1.5–3.5 \times 10^{9}/l$
Eosinophils $0–0.44 \times 10^{9}/l$
Monocytes $0.2–0.8 \times 10^{9}/l$
ESR (Westergren)
  male   3–5 mm/h
  female   4–10 mm/h
Prothrombin ratio (BCR)   1.0–1.3

Bleeding time (template)	3–10 min
Leukocyte alkaline phosphatase	15–60/100 leukocytes
Vitamin B_{12}	180–750 ng/l
Folate	2–14 µg/l
Fibrinogen degradation products (FDP)	<16 mg/l

Paper 1

Question 1.1

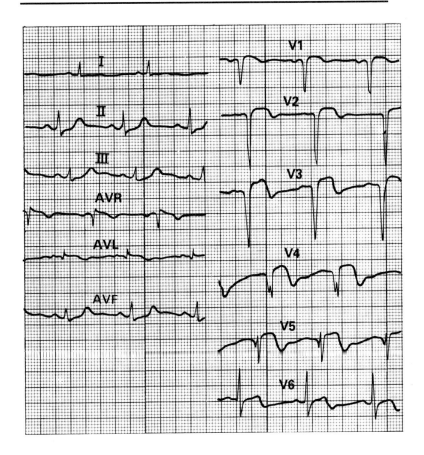

What is the diagnosis?

Answer to question 1.1

Recent anterior myocardial infarction

Deep Q waves, elevated ST segments and partial T wave
inversion are seen in V1–V5. These changes are
pathognomonic of recent anterior infarction. The early T
wave inversion suggests the infarct is between 3 and 7 days
old.

The notching of the QRS system in V4 and V5 is due to an
associated intraventricular conduction defect; not a bundle
branch block.

Question 1.2

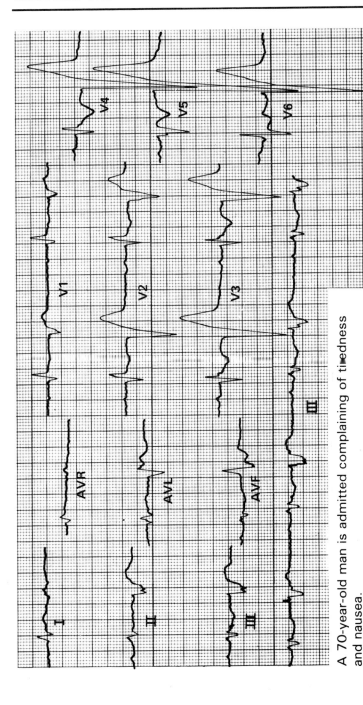

A 70-year-old man is admitted complaining of tiredness and nausea.

1. What abnormalities are present?
2. What is the cause of his symptoms?

Answer to question 1.2

1.a First degree heart block

The PR interval varies between 0.22 and 0.24 s. This is prolonged. The upper limit of normal is generally taken to be 0.22s.

b. Coupled ventricular ectopics (bigemini)

c. Old anterior myocardial infarction

In the sinus beats there is poor R wave progression in the chest leads.

d. Right bundle branch block

The QRS complex is prolonged (0.12 s) with an RSR pattern in V1–V4.

e. Digoxin effect

The ST segments slope downwards leading into an inverted T wave; the 'reversed tick' sign. This is seen in patients on cardiac glycosides but does not necessarily indicate toxicity. The change is best shown in the infero-lateral leads.

2.   Digoxin toxicity

Tiredness and nausea are both symptoms of digoxin toxicity. Other symptoms that may occur include anorexia and disturbances of colour vision of which xanthopsia is said to be the most characteristic. Bradycardia, first degree heart block and coupled ventricular ectopics are common features of digoxin toxicity although almost any arrhythmia may be seen.

Question 1.3

A 35-year-old woman with Crohn's disease is investigated
for anaemia:
Haemoglobin 8.0 g/dl
MCV 112 fl
Film: Macrocytosis + +
Serum B_{12} 80 ng/l

Schilling test	%Oral dose excreted in the urine
Part I (without intrinsic factor)	3.1%
Part II (with intrinsic factor)	3.5%
After 10 days of treatment with oxytetracycline repeat Part 1	11.4%

1. What is the underlying cause of her anaemia?
2. What other investigations are useful in making this
   diagnosis?

Answer to question 1.3

1. **Blind loop syndrome**
   She has a macrocytic anaemia due to Vitamin B_{12}
   deficiency. The causes of B_{12} deficiency are:
   a. **Absence of intrinsic factor**
      Due to intrinsic factor or gastric parietal cell
      antibodies—pernicious anaemia.
   b. **Disease of the terminal ileum** (the area where B_{12} is
      absorbed) eg. Crohn's disease, surgical resection.
   c. **Competition for B_{12} absorption**
      Blind loop syndrome.
      Fish tape worm.
   In the Schilling test 1 mg of radiolabelled B_{12} is given
   orally with a simultaneous injection of 1000 mg of
   cyanocobalamin. Urine is collected for 24 h and the
   percentage of absorbed B_{12} is calculated by measuring
   the proportion of the radiolabel that appears in the urine.
   If the amount is 5% or less there is significant
   malabsorption of B_{12}.
   In pernicious anaemia or following gastrectomy B_{12}
   malabsorption is corrected by intrinsic factor. In terminal
   ileal disease absorption remains impaired after either
   intrinsic factor or antibiotics.
   In blind loop syndrome (a common feature of Crohn's
   disease) overgrowth of bacteria occurs in parts of the
   bowel where there is stagnation of intestinal contents.
   This may occur in diverticula or in loops of bowel which
   have been bypassed either surgically or following the
   development of fistulae. The overgrowth of bacteria
   (usually anaerobes) compete for the absorption of B_{12}
   resulting in a deficiency of the vitamin. Oral tetracycline
   reduces the number of organisms and B_{12} absorption is
   returned to normal.

2. a. **Barium meal and follow through**
   b. **Urinary indican**
   c. **C^{14} Breath test**
   d. **Direct sampling and culture of intestinal contents**

Question 1.4

A fit, 36-year-old woman is referred for investigation of hypertension (BP 220/130). The physical examination was unremarkable. The only therapy she is taking is Captopril 25 mg t.d.s., prescribed by her GP.
Sodium 145 mmol/l
Potassium 3.2 mmol/l
Bicarbonate 34 mmol/l
Urea 5.6 mmol/l
There was a trace of glycosuria.

1. Suggest a diagnosis.
2. Give three relevant diagnostic investigations.

Answer to question 1.4

1. **Conn's syndrome**

   Primary hyperaldosteronism is a cause of hypertension in around 1% of patients, and is secondary to either an adrenal adenoma or adrenal hyperplasia. The diagnosis is suggested by the association of hypertension with hypokalaemia, the raised bicarbonate and a sodium over 140 mmol/l. Mild glucose intolerance is a rare association. The differential diagnosis includes Cushing's syndrome where diabetes is more common. There are no physical characteristics of Cushing's Syndrome and the hyperkalaemia is more severe than usual unless the Cushing's syndrome was secondary to ectopic ACTH production. Other possible diagnoses include liquorice or carbenoxalone administration, and causes of secondary hyperaldosteronism associated with hypertension. The hypertension is resistant to ACE inhibitors which provides further support for the diagnosis.

2. Raised aldosterone levels in the presence of low circulating renin will confirm the diagnosis. Selective venous catheterisation will enable lateralisation of the source of aldosterone, and arteriography or cholesterol scanning will provide further diagnostic information.

Question 1.5

A woman with a mastectomy scar complained of backache, bruising and fatigue. She has received no treatment.
Haemoglobin 10.7 g/dl
Platelets 50 × 10^9/l
Prothrombin time 26 s (control 12 s)
Kaolin cephalin clotting time 55 s (control 38 s)

1. What is the haematological diagnosis?
2. What other investigations would you do?

Answer to Question 1.5

1. **Disseminated intravascular coagulation (DIC)**
   This is probably due to carcinomatosis. The prolonged prothrombin time and Kaolin cephalin clotting time indicates deficiencies of more than one clotting factor. Combined with thrombocytopenia this suggests DIC. The haemostatic mechanism is inappropriately activated resulting in widespread fibrin formation and consumption of clotting factors and secondary platelet depletion. The fall in haemoglobin may be due to associated haemolysis produced by a microangiopathic haemolytic anaemia which is commonly associated with DIC in disseminated malignant disease. Evidence of secondary organ damage may be present, e.g. uraemia, skin necrosis etc. The process may be initiated by:
   a. Release of tissue thromboplastins
   b. Excessive endothelial damage

2. **Fibrin degradation products (FDP)**
   The fibrinolytic process is activated secondary to DIC producing increased circulating FDPs. There will also be low fibrinogen levels.

Question 1.6

A 25-year-old man with cervical lymphadenopathy
complains of generalised pruritus for 2 months.
Haemoglobin 6.0 g/dl
MCV 103 fl
MCHC 33 g/dl
WBC 8.0 × 10⁹/l
  Neutrophils 60%
  Eosinophils 15%
  Lymphocytes 20%
  Monocytes 5%
Film: Polychromasia + +
  Spherocytes +

1. What single diagnosis could explain the above?
2. Explain the anaemia.

Answer to question 1.6

1. **Hodgkin's disease**
   Lymphadenopathy, pruritus, eosinophilia and haemolytic anaemia (see below) strongly suggest a lymphoma. In a 25-year-old man Hodgkin's disease would be the most likely type.

2. **Haemolytic anaemia**
   The polychromasia and the raised MCV are due to an excess of reticulocytes in the peripheral blood. The causes of reticulocytes are:
   a. Haemolytic anaemia
   b. Following acute blood loss.
   In this case, haemolysis is supported by the presence of spherocytes. Hereditary spherocytosis would explain the haematological, but not the clinical findings. Hodgkin's disease is a recognised cause of acquired autoimmune haemolytic anaemia.

   Other causes of autoimmune haemolytic anaemia (AHA) include:
   a. Primary — idiopathic warm AHA
       — idiopathic chronic cold AHA
       — Evans syndrome
        (AHA + thrombocytopenia)
   b. Secondary — 'warm' antibodies
     — SLE + other autoimmune disorders
     — lymphoma especially CLL + Hodgkin's
     — drug-induced — Methyldopa
         — Levadopa
         — Mefenamic acid
     — carcinomatosis
   c. Secondary — 'cold' antibodies
     — histiocytic lymphoma
     — paroxysmal cold haemoglobinuria
     — infectious mononucleosis
     — mycoplasma pneumoniae infection

Question 1.7

A 27-year-old girl presented with an acute onset of
abdominal pain, muscle pains and symmetrical shoulder
weakness. The only medication she took was the oral
contraceptive.

Sodium   124 mmol/l
Potassium   4.8 mmol/l
Bilirubin   42 µmol/l
AST   45 iu/l

Ehrlichs test gave a pink colour which after the addition of
n-butanol remained in the lower aqueous phase.

1. What is the diagnosis?
2. What two other diagnostic tests should be performed?

Answer to question 1.7

1. **Acute intermittent porphyria**
   Abdominal pain is a common presenting symptom and when associated with neuropsychiatric symptoms an abnormality of porphyrin metabolism should be suspected. The clinical picture of other acute porphyrias is similar but cutaneous lesions are often present in porphyria variegata and hereditary coproporphyria is very rare. Acute intermittent porphyria usually presents after puberty and is commoner in women. It may be precipitated by a variety of drugs, including oral contraceptives. A raised bilirubin, transaminases and hyponatraemia are the commonest biochemical features although dehydration may occur following vomiting. Ehrlichs test gives a pink colour with porphobilinogen or with urobilinogen. The addition of n-butanol can distinguish between the two substances because porphobilinogen is insoluble in n-butanol (i.e. remains in the aqueous phase). Chloroform may be used instead of n-butanol but may give false +ve results.

2. Measurement of urinary δ-aminolaevulinic acid and urinary porphobilinogen, both of which are markedly increased in an attack of acute intermittent porphyria.

Question 1.8

A baby of 4 months with gastro-enteritis:
Sodium 155 mmol/l
Potassium 3.4 mmol/l
Urea 14.7 mmol/l

1. What two factors could have produced the
   hypenatraemia?
2. What is the first step in management of this baby?

Answer to question 1.8

1. a. **Intestinal water loss**
   In infantile gastro-enteritis the liquid stools have a low sodium content leading to predominant water deficiency resulting in haemoconcentration and hypernatraemia.
   b. **Feeding with full strength artificial feeds**
   Such foods are hypertonic. Water is lost in the stool and the solute is absorbed exacerbating the hypernatraemia. This complication is rare in breast fed babies because breast milk is less hypertonic. In contrast to conscious adults, babies are unable to say that they are thirsty. In consequence the mother may continue hypertonic fluids when water is required.

2. **Administration of hypotonic fluids**
   Convulsions and permanent cerebral damage can occur in hypernatraemic dehydration. The sodium level should be lowered and the water replaced by the administration of low solute fluids either orally or slowly intravenously. If the infusion is too rapid, cerebral haemorrhage may result.

Question 1.9

Cardiac catheter results on a woman of 45:

Chamber	Pressure (mmHg)
Right atrium	30/15
Right ventricle	70/15
Pulmonary artery	70/40
End diastolic pulmonary artery wedge	35
Left ventricle	105/5
Aorta	100/70

Give the cardiac diagnoses.

Answer to question 1.9

1. Mitral stenosis
There is an end diastolic pressure gradient of 30 mmHg across the mitral valve which is highly significant, indicating stenosis. A measurable end diastolic gradient is abnormal.

2. Pulmonary hypertension
A pulmonary artery systolic pressure of 70 mmHg (NR: 20–30) signifies pulmonary hypertension, in this case secondary to mitral stenosis.

3. Right ventricular overload
The right ventricular end diastolic pressure is normally less than 5 mmHg. The raised pressure (15 mmHg) reflects overload resulting from pulmonary hypertension.

4. Tricuspid regurgitation
The maximum pressure, or systolic wave, in the right atrium is very high. A pressure this high only occurs in tricuspid valve disease. As the atrial diastolic pressure is equal to the right ventricular end diastolic pressure, the lesion is probably tricuspid incompetence without stenosis. This could be functional, i.e. dilatation of the valve ring, or due to intrinsic rheumatic valve disease.

Question 1.10

A 15-year-old boy presents with failure to develop
secondary sexual characteristics.
Height 151 cm (NR 3rd–97th centile 156–181 cm)
LH 6.0 iu/l
FSH 3.9 iu/l
Testosterone 8 nmol/l

After an intravenous injection of 100 μg of gonadotrophin
releasing hormone (LHRH)
LH 38.1 iu/l
FHS 7.5 iu/l

1. What is the diagnosis?
2. What other investigation is indicated?
3. What management would you recommend?

Answer to question 1.10

1. **Constitutional delayed puberty**

   Puberty is delayed if secondary sexual development does not begin by age 14 in boys. He has an unusually short stature for his chronoligical age (less than the 3rd centile). The differential diagnosis includes constitutionally delayed puberty, hypogonadotrophic hypogonadism and hypergonadotrophic hypogonadism. The serum testosterone in all three will be low (at prepubertal levels). The low (prepubertal) values of gonadotrophins excludes hypergonadotrophic hypogonadism, e.g. Klinefelter's syndrome, primary testicular failure etc.

   In this case the LH response to gonadotrophin releasing hormone is pubertal (a rise of >16 iu/l), suggesting that secondary sexual development will commence within six months. There is frequently a family history of delayed puberty.

2. **Bone age**

   A wrist bone age score should be appropriate for stature (i.e. delayed).

3. Clinical observation for signs of pubertal development and measurement of the rise in testosterone, as well as appropriate psychological support. A course of human chorionic gonadotrophin injection may be used to induce puberty. Continuous treatment with testosterone is not indicated as it may compromise final height and skeletal development.

Paper 2

Question 2.1

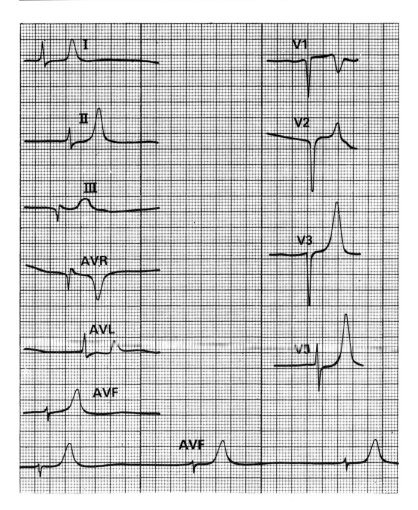

A 54-year-old becomes drowsy and confused. This is her ECG.

1. What abnormalities are present?
2. What is the diagnosis?
3. What would be your first therapeutic measure?

Answer to question 2.1

1. The following abnormalities are present:
   a. Profound bradycardia rate 30/min
   b. Absent P waves.
   c. Q waves in V1 and V2 suggesting old anterior infarction.
   d. Tall, tented T waves.
   The prolonged QT interval (0.46 s) is consistent with this degree of bradycardia.

2. Hyperkalaemia
   All the features listed above with the exception of **c** are typical ECG findings. The potassium was 8.4 mmol/1.

3. Intravenous calcium
   10 mls of 10% calcium gluconate or calcium chloride given by slow intravenous injection will reverse the ECG abnormalities and help prevent asystole.
   Other measures useful in hyperkalaemia:
   a. i.v. Dextrose and insulin.
   b. Rectal resonium — the rectal route is far more effective than the oral route as the rectal mucosa contains more exchangeable potassium.
   c. Dialysis.
   d. i.v. Bicarbonate may be used with extreme care.

Question 2.2

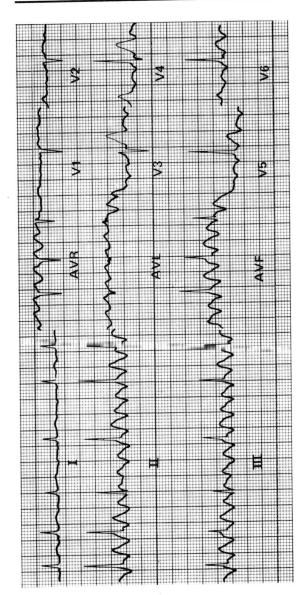

Routine ECG on a 66-year-old man with an irregular pulse.

1. What abnormality is present?
2. Give the three most likely causes

Answer to question 2.2

1. **Atrial flutter with variable block**
   Atrial rate 300, mean ventricular rate approximately 100.
   Atrial activity is represented by the characteristic 'saw
   tooth' (wide, large voltage) waves, sometimes called
   flutter waves. In this case they are best seen in leads II, III
   and AVF. They are completely regular. The QRS
   complexes are irregularly spaced indicating variable
   degrees of conduction through the AV node. The QRS
   complex shows a varying conduction pattern and this is
   best seen in lead III.

2. **Ischaemic heart disease**
   Particularly following myocardial infarction.
   Digoxin therapy
   Mitral valve disease
   Other causes include:
   Hypertensive heart disease
   Atrial septal defect
   sick sinus syndrome
   alcoholic cardiomyopathy
   Other general causes of tachycardia (e.g. fever,
   thyrotoxicosis, tricylic antidepressant overdose) may be
   associated with atrial flutter in predisposed individuals.

Question 2.3

A 19-year-old girl with asthma is admitted with dyspnoea.
She is given 28% oxygen by the casualty staff. Her
dyspnoea worsens after aminophylline 250 mg i.v.
Sodium 137 mmol/1
Potassium 4.7 mmol/1
Arterial blood gases:
pH 7.65
pCO_2 2.5 kPa
pO_2 21.5 kPa
Bicarbonate 21 mmol/1

1. What is the diagnosis?
2. How would you treat this girl?

Answer to question 2.3

1. **Hysterical overbreathing**
   The classical features of an acute respiratory alkalosis are present, namely high pH and low pCO_2. There has been insufficient time for plasma bicarbonate to drop through urinary excretion.
   Causes of respiratory alkalosis
   Hysteria
   Salicylates (in association with metabolic acidosis)
   Brain stem lesions + raised intracranial pressure
   Excessive artificial ventilation

2. **Reassurance**
   In this case overbreathing followed the correction of bronchospasm with aminophylline. Sympathetic handling was enough to relieve her apparent dyspnoea.
   Alternative measures such as re-breathing or sedation should not be used except with extreme caution in an asthmatic.

Question 2.4

A 35-year-old patient who has been on haemodialysis for
10 years complains of bone pain. He has been on no drugs
except for aluminium hydroxide tablets.
Pre-dialysis results:
Calcium 3.5 mmol/l
Phosphate 0.6 mmol/l
Alkaline phosphatase 350 iu/l

1. What is the most likely diagnosis?
2. What treatment would correct the disorder?

Answer to question 2.4

1. **Tertiary hyperparathyroidism**
   The patient is hypercalcaemic with a high alkaline phosphatase and a low phosphate. The level of phosphate varies in renal failure, being influenced by:
   a. Dialysis
   b. Diet
   c. Treatment with aluminium hydroxide — which forms insoluble aluminium phosphate in the gut, thus preventing phosphate absorption
   d. Parathormone levels
   Secondary hyperparathyroidism is common in long standing renal failure, and results from hypocalcaemia. In secondary hyperparathyroidism parathormone secretion remains appropriate to the level of calcium. However, after prolonged feedback stimulation, parathormone secretion may become autonomous and lead to hypercalcaemia.
   The raised alkaline phosphatase is due to the associated bone disease. Tertiary hyperparathyroidism is not uncommon in patients on long-term haemodialysis.

2. **Subtotal parathyroidectomy,** or removal of the parathyroid adenoma if present.

Question 2.5

A 60-year-old man with vitiligo presents with tiredness
and paraesthesiae.
Haemoglobin 6.0 g/dl
MCV 112 fl
MCHC 34 g/dl
WBC 3.9 $\times$ 10^9/l
Platelets 80 $\times$ 10^9/l
Bilirubin 40 μmol/l
AST 20 iu/l
Alkaline phosphatase 55 iu/l

1. What is the most likely diagnosis?
2. Name three further tests necessary to confirm this
   diagnosis.

Answer to question 2.5

1. **Pernicious anaemia**
   There are four features:
   a. Vitiligo — see below
   b. Macrocytic anaemia
   c. Paraesthesiae suggesting peripheral nerve damage
   d. Mildly raised bilirubin in the presence of normal liver function tests, suggesting low grade haemolysis.

2. a. **Bone marrow**
   This would be hypercellular in most cases and show megaloblastic change, with other morphological abnormalities.
   b. **Serum B_{12}**
   This will be low.
   c. **Schilling or dicopac test**
   This will establish the aetiology of the vitamin B_{12} deficiency (see p. 8).

Question 2.6

A 36-year-old woman of Cushingoid appearance was
referred from a private psychiatric clinic. The following
investigations were performed:
Sodium 142 mmol/l
Potassium 3.8 mmol/l
Urea 1.9 mmol/l
AST 52 iu/l
Bilirubin 20 µmol/l
Alkaline phosphatase 150 iu/l
24 h urine cortisol excretion 400 nmol/l (NR $\leq$ 275)
Morning cortisol 280 nmol/l (after 1 mg dexamethasone
given at 10 pm)
Insulin tolerance test (0.25 unit/kg)

Time (min)	Blood glucose (mmol/l)	Cortisol (nmoml/l)
0	7.9	450
30	3.6	480
60	1.8	840
90	5.9	950
120	9.6	780

1. What two diagnoses are suggested by this data?
2. What advice would you give the patient and the
   psychiatrist?

Answer to question 2.6

1. **Alcoholic pseudocushing's and probable diabetes mellitus**

   This patient was under treatment for alcoholism and depression, both of which may be associated with the biochemical and physical features of Cushing's syndrome. The low urea and abnormal liver function tests are compatible with alcoholism. The three investigations presented are all screening tests for Cushing's disease. An elevated 24 h urinary cortisol excretion, and a failure of the plasma cortisol to suppress below 200 nmol/l after an overnight dexamethasone test are suggestive of Cushing's syndrome. When there is doubt about the diagnosis an insulin tolerance test will provide more information. In Cushing's syndrome the plasma cortisol fails to rise in response to adequate hypoglycaemia, because the inappropriately high cortisol levels suppress the stress response to hypoglycaemia. In pseudocushing's the normal response is preserved and a rise of more than 220 nmol/l in the plasma cortisol is expected. Adequate hypoglycaemia ($\leq$2.2 mmol/l) may be difficult to achieve because of insulin resistance. The fasting blood glucose is diagnostic of diabetes mellitus if measured in venous blood, but only 0.1 mmol above the cut off value if venous plasma is used for the estimation. A confirmatory value should be obtained before this diagnosis is confirmed.

2. The biochemical features of pseudocushing's will regress following 1–2 weeks alcohol abstention. No further management is necessary.

Question 2.7

A 65-year-old woman treated for hypertension for 20 years complains of tiredness and shortness of breath:
Haemoglobin 8.0 g/dl
MCV 98 fl
Film: Polychromasia
        Spherocytosis

1. What is the probable diagnosis?
2. What two tests would confirm it?

Answer to question 2.7

1. **Methyldopa-induced haemolytic anaemia**
   The polychromasia and raised MCV is due to an excess of
   reticulocytes. Although there are many other causes for
   anaemia with a reticulocytosis the history of longstanding
   treatment for hypertension should give the correct
   diagnosis. Approximately 20% of patients on methyldopa
   therapy for more than 1 year develop a positive Coombs'
   test, but overt signs of haemolysis occur in less than 1%.
   An IgG autoantibody against normal red cell membranes
   appears after 3–6 months treatment and remains for up
   to six months after treatment has been stopped although
   haemolysis ceases rapidly.

2. a. **Reticulocyte count**
   b. **Coombs' test.**

Question 2.8

A 38-year-old man complains of night sweats and
dizziness on standing.
Haemoglobin 9.6 g/dl
MCV 84 fl
WBC 5.2 × 10^9/l
   Polymorphs 45%
   Lymphocytes 53%
   Monocytes 2%
ESR 80 mm/h
Urea 7.6 mmol/l
Sodium 129 mmol/l
Potassium 5.8 mmol/l
Random blood glucose 3.2 mmol/l
MSU
   WBC — 250 × 10^6/l
   RBC — 0
   Film — no organisms
   Culture — no growth

1 What are the likeliest underlying conditions?
2. What investigations would you perform?

Answer to question 2.8

1. **Tuberculosis and Addison's disease**
   He has a normocytic anaemia with a high ESR. The
   electrolyte abnormalities and low blood sugar are
   suggestive of Addison's disease. (Primary adrenocortical
   deficiency). These findings combined with sterile pyuria
   suggest tuberculosis involving the renal tract.
   Chronic pyelonephritis could produce the same urinary
   and electrolyte findings, but would not explain the very
   raised ESR, and the low blood sugar.

2. a. **Short synacthen stimulation test**
      250 µg of tetracosactrin is given intramuscularly and
      blood for cortisol taken at 0, 30 (and 60) min. Failure
      of cortisol to rise by more than 250 nmol/l to a level
      of 550 nmol/l at 30 min is indicative of
      hypoadrenalism, and a normal response excludes
      primary adrenal failure.
   b. **Plain X-ray of the abdomen**
      This may show renal or adrenal calcification.
   c. **IVU**
      To assess the extent of renal involvement.
   d. **Early morning urine** for culture of acid fast bacilli.

Question 2.9

A boy aged two months is investigated for failure to gain weight and vomiting. He has hypospadias.
Sodium 126 mmol/l
Potassium 5.9 mmol/l
Bicarbonate 18 mmol/l
Urea 14.5 mmol/l
Creatinine 76 µmol/l
Glucose 2.6 mmol/l
Urinary sodium 62 mmol/l

1. What is the most likely diagnosis?
2. What other investigations are indicated?

Answer to question 2.9

1. **Congenital adrenal hyperplasia**
   There are features of mineralocorticoid and glucocorticoid deficiency. The most common enzyme deficiency is 21 hydroxylase, which is necessary to synthesise cortisol and aldosterone. If the defect is complete, salt wasting occurs, with high urinary sodium excretion leading to dehydration, vomiting, etc.

2. Measurement of 17 hydroxy-progesterone, which is the substrate for the defective enzyme, will enable rapid confirmation of the diagnosis. The genitalia may be ambiguous, with masculinisation of the female, due to excessive androgen production, producing clitoral enlargement and labial fusion. This may be confused with a male who has cryptorchidism and hypospadias. The sex of the infant should be confirmed by a buccal smear and karyotype.

Question 2.10

A 65-year-old lady complains of thirst, nocturia and a
thyroid mass.
Sodium 135 mmol/l
Potassium 4.2 mmol/l
Calcium 2.86 mmol/l
Phosphate 0.92 mmol/l
Albumin 40 g/l
Alkaline phosphatase 80 iu/l
Glucose 6.7 mmol/l
TSH 18 mu/l

1. What is the diagnosis?
2. What is the treatment?

Answer to question 2.10

1. **Primary hypothyroidism**
   The TSH is elevated indicating primary hypothyroidism.
   There is a rare association between Hashimoto's
   thyroiditis and hypercalcaemia produced by the
   diminished incorporation of calcium into bone.

2. The treatment is thyroid replacement therapy with
   thyroxine. The serum calcium will return to normal.

   Association of a thyroid mass and hypercalcaemia.
   a. Hashimoto's thyroiditis.
   b. Follicular carcinoma of thyroid with bone secondaries.
   c. Medullary carcinoma of thyroid is associated with
      hyperparathyroidism in the multiple endocrine
      adenoma syndrome type II (Sipple's syndrome).

Paper 3

Question 3.1

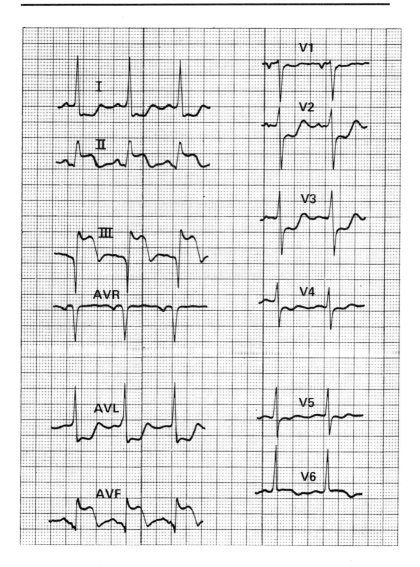

A 54-year-old woman presents with a syncopal attack associated with sweating.

1. What is the diagnosis?
2. How recent is the cardiac lesion?

Answer to question 3.1

1. **Inferior myocardial infarction**
   The features are:
   a. Pathological Q waves in III and AVF.
   b. ST elevation in II, III and AVF.
   c. Early T wave inversion II, III, AVF and V6.
   d. Reciprocal ST depression in I, AVL, V1–V5.

2. **Less than three days**
   The dominant abnormality is the ST elevation. If the lesion were older T wave changes would be more prominent.
   The order of appearance of ECG changes in myocardial infarction is as follows:
   a. ST elevation: 1–6 hours
   b. Q waves: approximately 24 h
   c. T wave changes: 2–7 days
   The order of disappearance:
   a. ST elevation (persistance suggests the possibility of a ventricular aneurysm)
   b. T wave inversion.
   c. Q waves. These are usually permanent.

Question 3.2

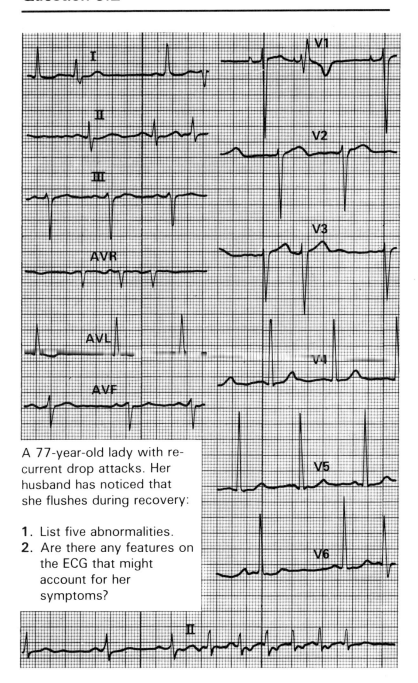

A 77-year-old lady with re-current drop attacks. Her husband has noticed that she flushes during recovery:

1. List five abnormalities.
2. Are there any features on the ECG that might account for her symptoms?

Answer to question 3.2

1. a. Left ventricular hypertrophy
   The height of the R wave in V5 plus the depth of the S
   wave in V2 exceeds 35 mm. (Sokolow's criteria).
   Although Sokolow's criteria of LVH are met, LVH is
   not present if the point system devised by Romhilt and
   Estes is used.

b. Left axis deviation (LAD)
   The axis is approximately $-30°$. The most commonly
   used normal range lies between 0 and $+90°$. If the
   axis lies beyond $-30°$ unequivocal LAD is present.

c. Atrial ectopics
   Some show a pattern of aberrant conduction, eg. the
   ectopics in V_1 which is preceded by a P wave, shows
   RBBB pattern and has therefore been conducted by the
   left bundle.

d. A short run of atrial tachycardia
   Seen in lead II. The rate is approximately 170 per min.

2.   Yes — atrial tachycardia
   The history is typical of syncope due to an arrhythmia.
   In this patient atrial tachycardia has been
   demonstrated and could be responsible for her
   symptoms. If there was an underlying sick sinus
   syndrome, other arrhythmias, eg. sinus arrest, sinus
   bradycardia, might be demonstrated on a 24-h ECG
   tape.

Question 3.3

A man of 50 presents with recurrent faints. He has an abdominal surgical scar.

Hb. 9.2 g/dl
MCV 73 fl   *Fe def*
MCHC 24 g/dl
75 gram glucose tolerance test:
Blood glucose 0 hours 6.0 mmol/l
$\frac{1}{2}$ hour 13.0 mmol/l   *lag curve*
1 hour 10.5 mmol/l   *post gastrectomy*
$1\frac{1}{2}$ hour 2.1 mmol/l
2 hours 3.0 mmol/l

Give an explanation for these findings.

Answer to question 3.3

Previous partial gastrectomy and **dumping syndrome**
There is a hypochromic microcytic anaemia typical of iron
deficiency. This is a recognised late complication of partial
gastrectomy, due to intestinal hurry and failure to absorb
iron. In addition there is a lag storage GTT with late
hypoglycaemia responsible for his faints.

Complications of gastric surgery
Mechanical:
   early dumping
   late dumping
   afferent loop syndrome
   diarrhoea
   intestinal hurry with malabsorption
Nutritional:
   iron dificiency anaemia
   B_{12} deficiency (intrinsic factor deficiency)
   osteomalacia
   osteoporosis
Stomal ulcer
Operative complications — wound infection,
                               pneumonia, etc.

Causes of lag storage GTT
Gastric surgery
Thyrotoxicosis
Severe liver disease
Early diabetes mellitus
Some normal subjects

Question 3.4

A 42-year-old woman gives a three year history of
recurrent renal colic. She complains of 'gritty' eyes:
Calcium 3.22 mmol/l
Phosphate 0.60 mmol/l
Alkaline phosphatase 111 iu/l
Albumin 41 g/l
Urea 8.2 mmol/l
After hydrocortisone 40 mg t.d.s. for ten days
Calcium 2.95 mmol/l
Albumin 38 g/l

What is the diagnosis?

Answer to question 3.4

Primary hyperparathyroidism
There are the following features:

1. **Hypercalcaemia** which fails to suppress (ie. fall to within the normal range) with corticosteroids. This occurs in:
   primary and tertiary hyperparathyroidism
   Severe thyrotoxicosis
   Some cases of malignant disease.
   The slight fall in the calcium after hydrocortisone is in part due to fluid retention, which is reflected in the lowered serum albumin.

2. **Hypophosphataemia.** Hypercalcaemia with hypophosphataemia is only seen in primary and tertiary hyperparathyroidism and ectopic parathormone secretion, because of excess circulating parathyroid hormone.

3. A raised alkaline phosphatase which suggests established bone disease. The length of the history (three years) suggests that primary hyperparathyroidism is the most likely diagnosis. The 'gritty' eyes are due to corneal calcification.

Question 3.5

A 64-year-old man presents to Outpatients with lassitude.
He has received no therapy.
Haemoglobin 7.9 g/dl
MCV 84 fl
MCHC 31 g/dl
Film: Dimorphic picture of normochromic and hypochromic
cells
Reticulocytes 4%
WBC 4.2 $\times$ 10^9/l
  neutrophils 65%
  lymphocytes 35%
Platelets 227 $\times$ 10^9/l

1. What is the diagnosis?
2. How is the diagnosis confirmed?
3. What medication may be useful?
4. Give three possible underlying causes.

Answer to question 3.5

1. Sideroblastic anaemia
He has a normochromic normocytic anaemia with a dimorphic film. The types of dimorphism are:

a. Mixed hypochromic and normochromic, seen in sideroblastic anaemia and partially treated iron deficiency anaemia.

b. Mixed macrocytic and microcytic which may be found in patients with iron deficiency together with B_{12} or folate deficiency. Blood transfusion may cause a dimorphic picture where there is a morphological difference between the cells of the donor and the recipient.

2. Marrow aspiration
The diagnosis of sideroblastic anaemia is confirmed by the finding of ring sideroblasts in the bone marrow. These are red cell precursors with cytoplasmic iron granules forming a ring round the nucleus.

3. Pyridoxine
Both the primary and the secondary form may respond (approximately 30%).

4. Possible causes include:
Hereditary sex-linked
Acquired:

a. Primary or idiopathic

b. Secondary:

    (i) **Toxic**
        Alcohol
        Lead
        Antituberculous drugs

    (ii) **Dyshaemopoetic**
        Myeloproliferative disorders
        Haemolytic anaemia
        Megaloblastic anaemia
        Collagenoses—particularly RA
        Carcinoma

Question 3.6

A baby has had three fits, each occurring early in the
morning. He is noted to have hepatomegaly.
Fasting blood glucose 2.2 mmol/l
AST (SGOT) 18 iu/l
Bilirubin 13 µmol/l
Alkaline phosphatase 360 iu/l
Urate 0.78 mmol/l

1. What is the cause of the fits?
2. What is the diagnosis?
3. How is the diagnosis confirmed?
4. Comment on the alkaline phosphatase level.

Answer to question 3.6

1. **Hypoglycaemia.**
   The tendency for the fits to occur in the early morning is related to the period of relative starvation which occurs overnight. The causes of infantile hypoglycaemia are:
   a. **Idiopathic hypoglycaemia** — this probably represents a mixture of different metabolic abnormalities where specific enzyme deficiencies have not been defined.
   b. **Leucine hypersensitivity** — foods containing leucine, particularly casein, which is found in milk products, may precipitate hypoglycaemia in affected individuals in the first six months of life.
   c. **Glycogen storage diseases** — this group consists of a number of diseases each characterised by a deficiency of enzymes responsible for glycogenolysis. Hence it accumulates in the liver causing hepatomegaly.
   d. **Hereditary fructose intolerance** — the defect causes an accumulation of fructose-1-phosphate which is thought to inhibit glycogenolysis and gluconeogenesis.
   e. **Insulinomas** — these occur, but are extremely rare in infancy.
   f. **Babies of diabetic mothers** may be hypoglycaemic in the neonatal period, due to fetal islet cell hyperlasia induced during intrauterine life.

2. **Von Gierke's disease** (Type I glycogen storage disease). The presence of hepatomegaly suggests a storage disease and the raised uric acid occurs only in type I. There is a deficiency of glucose-6-phosphatase.
3. **By demonstrating deficiency of the enzyme in a liver biopsy.** The glucagon test or galactose infusion test may also be used.
4. **It is normal for a growing child.**

Question 3.7

A 35-year-old lady with backache. X-rays show collapse
of D8:
Haemoglobin 11.5 g/dl
MCV 69 gl
MCHC 24 g/dl
WBC 4.5 × 10⁹/l
Film: right shift of neutrophils
Urea 2.4 mmol/l
Calcium 1.75 mmol/l
Phosphate 0.8 mmol/l
Alkaline phosphatase 210 iu/l
Albumin 28 g/l

1. Why is the calcium low?
2. Explain the vertebral fracture.

Answer to question 3.7

1. Malabsorption

Apart from the low calcium there are the following features of malabsorption:

a. Hypochromic microcytic anaemia, suggesting iron deficiency.

b. A right shift of neutrophils compatible with B_{12} or folate deficiency.

c. Hypoalbuminaemia.

d. The low normal urea.

Other causes of hypocalcaemia include:

Hypoparathyroidism

Pseudohypoparathyroidism

Calcium and vitamin D deficiency

Chronic renal failure

Hypoalbuminaemia (including haemodilution)

Hypoparathyroidism, pseudohypoparathyroidism and chronic renal failure are characteristically associated with a raised, not low serum phosphate. In hypoalbuminaemia the calcium will fall in direct proportion to the albumin, but in this case the corrected calcium is significantly below the lower limit of normal.

2. Osteomalacia associated with hypocalcaemia

The low serum phosphate with the low calcium is typical of calcium and vitamin D deficiency. The raised alkaline phosphatase, due to osteoblastic overactivity, indicates the presence of osteomalacia, which is also manifested in this case by the spontaneous fracture.

Question 3.8

A 52-year-old man complains of breathlessness.
Forced vital capacity (FVC) 1.8 l
FEV_1 1.45 l
Resting transfer factor 17 ml min^{-1} $mmHg^{-1}$
Haemoglobin 11.2 g/dl
ESR 76 mm/hr
Rheumatoid factors: Sheep cell aggulination titre
                       (SCAT) 1/512
                       Latex 1/2560
Anti-nuclear factor (ANF) 1/8
DNA binding 12 units (NR<25 units)

1. What is the underlying disease?
2. What is the cause of his breathlessness?

Answer to question 3.8

1. Rheumatoid arthritis (RA)

There is a strongly positive rheumatoid factor and the presence of ANF is a common finding in RA, but the low titre of ANF and the normal DNA binding is strong evidence against systemic lupus erythematosus.

2. Pulmonary fibrosis

There is a low vital capacity with a normal FEV_1/FVC ratio, i.e. a restrictive defect. This is a recognised complication of RA occurring in 2–5% of cases. It is commoner in male patients with nodules and is associated with a high titre of rheumatoid factor.

Question 3.9

A 64-year-old man presents with hepatosplenomegaly,
lymphadenopathy and retinal haemorrhages:
Haemoglobin 11.0 g/dl
WBC 3.7 × 10⁹/l
    Neutrophils 50%
    Lymphocytes 35%
    Monocytes 10%
    Eosinophils 5%
Platelets 105 × 10⁹/l
ESR 110 mm/h
Total protein 90g/l
IgG 1.2 g/l
IgA 0.8 g/l
IgM 16.8 g/l
Urine for Bence–Jones protein-positive.

1. What is the diagnosis?
2. Give a likely cause for the retinal haemorrhages.
3. What cell type will predominate in the marrow?

Answer to question 3.9

1. Waldenströms macroglobulinaemia

There is a high total protein level of which a substantial proportion is IgM. A rise in IgM of this order (10 times the upper limit of normal) is only found in malignant paraproteinaemias. The low levels of IgG and IgA indicate an associated immune paresis. The very high ESR reflects the hyperglobulinaemia. The slight reduction in haemoglobin, white count and platelets suggest hypersplenism or marrow involvement. Bence–Jones proteinuria is a recognised but unusual feature of this disease, occuring in about 10% of patients. High levels of monoclonal IgM may be very rarely found in chronic lymphocytic leukaemia and some lymphomas.

2. Hyperviscosity syndrome

The high protein concentration may increase the blood's viscosity, causing slowing of the micro-circulation and sludging in the capillaries. This is said to be the cause of the marked haemorrhagic tendency that is a feature of this disease. Thrombocytopenia, impaired platelet function and inhibition of clotting factors may contribute to a bleeding tendency.

3. Lymphocytes

In contrast to myeloma where plasma cells may be increased, Waldenström's macroglobulinaemia is characterised by an increase in lymphocytes in the marrow. A small proportion of these may show an increase in cytoplasm (plasmacytoid lymphocytes) which may be PAS positive, a finding of important diagnostic significance.

Question 3.10

A 55–year–old man collapses outside a restaurant with a fit. He was on no drug therapy.
Sodium 115 mmol/l
Potassium 3.8 mmol/l
Urea 1.8 mmol/l
Total protein 52 g/l
Urine osmolality 450 mosm/kg

1. What is the underlying endocrine abnormality?
2. What test should be done to confirm your diagnosis?
3. How would you initially treat this man?

Answer to question 3.10

1. **Inappropriate ADH secretion**
   There are two features of haemodilution:
   a. Low urea and total protein
   b. Hyponatraemia
   The causes of haemodilution are:
   a. Inappropriate ADH syndrome, which may present as epilepsy, which in this case was the cause of the patient's collapse
   b. Water overload (including psychogenic polydipsia)
   c. Salt depletion, e.g. loss from vomit, diarrhoea, fistulae and sweating, with replacement with hypotonic fluid
   d. Renal failure
   e. Hypothyroidism

2. **Plasma and urinary osmolality**
   In inappropirate ADH secretion plasma osmolality is low and urinary osmolality high.

3. **Restrict water** intake, then treat the underlying cause.

   The causes of inappropriate ADH secretion are:
   a. Malignancy:
      Oat cell carcinoma of the bronchus
      Carcinoma of the pancreas
      Hodgkin's disease
   b. Following head injury
   c. Infections:
      Meningitis
      Pneumonia and other severe pulmonary infections
      Pulmonary tuberculosis
   d. Drugs:
      Chlorpromazine
      Carbamazepine
   e. Acute intermittent porphyria

Paper 4

Question 4.1

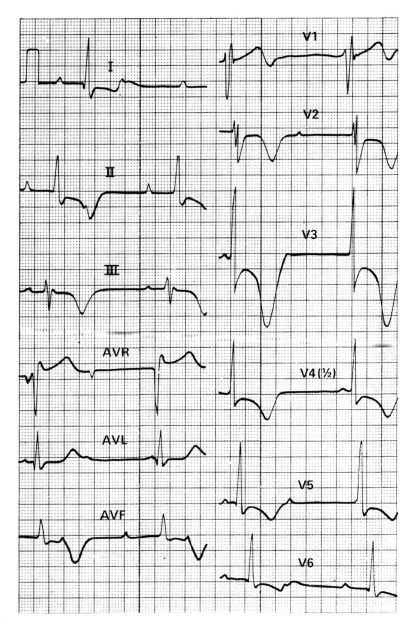

What abnormalities are present on this ECG?

Answer to question 4.1

1. **Complete heart block**
   The atria and the ventricles are beating entirely
   independently of one another. The atrial rate is a regular
   75/min and the ventricular rate 36/min and regular. The
   QRS complex duration is greater than 0.12 s suggesting
   the ventricular pacemaker is distal to the bundle of His (a
   slow idioventricular rhythm) although the presence of a
   bundle branch block cannot be excluded.

2. **Giant 'T' wave inversion**
   This occurs in about 5% of patients with complete heart
   block and does not necessarily imply myocardial
   infarction.

Question 4.2

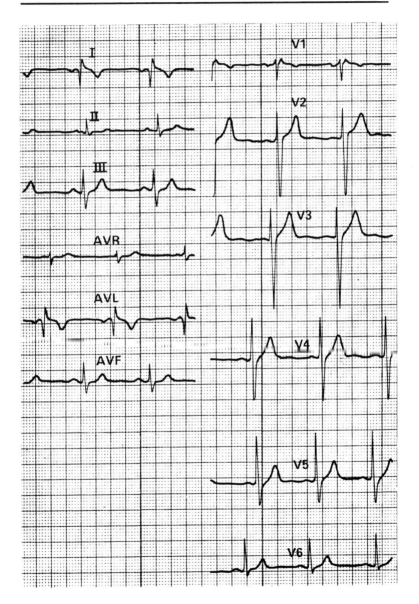

A 29-year-old man presents to casualty with chest pain at
2 a.m.
How do you account for the ECG findings?

Answer to question 4.2

The arm leads have been reversed

The clues are:

1. Isoelectric complexes in leads I and III with a positive in lead II. This combination is impossible if the leads were correctly connected.

2. An inverted PQRST in lead I. This is the mirror image of a normal tracing for this lead (right arm to left arm).

3. Apart from incomplete right bundle branch block, (a common innocent finding), the chest leads are normal.

Question 4.3

Catheter blood gases in a 25-year-old man:

Chamber	Oxygen saturation (%)
Right atrium	67
Right ventricle	65
Pulmonary artery	70
Left atrium	85
Left ventricle	78
Aorta	79

1. What is the diagnosis?
2. Is surgery indicated?

Answer to question 4.3

1. **Ventricular septal defect (VSD) with a right to left shunt, i.e. Eisenmenger's syndrome**
   Blood on the right side of the heart has a low PO_2 and left atrial blood has been oxygenated in its transit through the lungs. However, left ventricular blood is at a lower oxygen tension, indicating that dilution with hypoxic blood has occurred. There is, therefore, a right to left shunt at ventricular level.
   Initially in VSD the shunt is from left to right. This overloads the pulmonary circulation leading in time to pulmonary hypertension. Ultimately, right ventricular pressure exceeds left ventricular pressure and the shunt reverses.

2. **No**
   Once established a right to left shunt provides an outlet for blood from the right heart. Closure of the defect removes this safety valve and the pressure in the right heart rises, precipitating right ventricular failure, which is usually fatal.

Question 4.4

An obese 71-year-old non insulin dependent diabetic woman, recently bereaved, becomes acutely ill. She smells strongly of alcohol.

Haemoglobin	13.2 g/dl
WBC	$11 \times 10^9/l$
Sodium	141 mmol/l
Potassium	5.4 mmol/l
Chloride	88 mmol/l
Bicarbonate	7 mmol/l
Urea	9 mmol/l
Glucose	12.3 mmol/l
Urine	glucose 1%
	ketones — trace

141 + 54 = 146 4
88 + 7 = 95 + H⁻
51
netos acidosis

1. What is the metabolic diagnosis?
2. What are the three principal differential diagnoses?
3. What three investigations should be performed?

Answer to question 4.4

1. **Lactic acidosis**

   She has a profound metabolic acidosis manifested by the low bicarbonate and a high anion gap. The anion gap is calculated as follows:

   $$(Na^+ + K^+) - (Cl^- + HCO_{3^-}) =$$
   $$(141 + 5.4) - (88 + 7) \qquad = 51$$

   The upper limit of normal is 16–20 mmol/l. Metabolic acidosis with a high anion gap are due to ingestion or endogenous production of organic acids whose anions are not routinely measured.

   These anions may be:
   - **a.** Lactate
   - **b.** Ketoacids
   - **c.** Other organic acids, e.g. formate, oxalate, sulphates, phosphates
   - **d.** Salicylate

2. The differential diagnosis in a metabolic acidosis with a high anion gap include:
   - **a.** Biguanide therapy. Lactic acidosis is a complication of biguanide therapy in diabetics, especially those with cardiovascular, renal or hepatic disease. Phenformin is no longer used but there is still a slight risk of lactic acidosis with metformin.
   - **b.** Alcohol induced lactic acidosis. There is an accumulation of ketoacids and lactate. This is a rare complication of acute ethanol ingestion where the ethanol inhibits gluconeogenesis from a lactate substrate.
   - **c.** A high salicylate overdose may induce a high anion gap acidosis with accumulation of salicylate, lactate and ketoacids.

     This is not diabetic ketoacidosis (another high anion gap acidosis) because heavy ketonuria and dehydration are absent.

3. **a. Blood gases** to confirm metabolic acidosis.
   - **b. Blood salicylate levels** to exclude an Aspirin overdose.
   - **c. Blood lactate levels** to confirm the diagnosis. Blood lactate levels are normally less than 1 mmol/l.

Question 4.5

A 55-year-old woman complains to her GP of a 'dragging in the stomach'. On finding massive splenomegaly he performs a blood count.

Haemoglobin 9.6 g/dl
MCV 90 fl
Nucleated RBC 4/100 — red cells show
                        tear-drop poikilocytes
WBC 11.5 × 10⁹/l
      Neutrophils 60%
      Myelocytes 6%
      Metamyelocytes 2%
      Myeloblasts 1%
      Lymphocytes 31%
Platelets 650 × 10⁹/l

1. What is the haematological process?
2. What is the likely diagnosis?

↓ folate
↑ VitB12
↑ urate
↑ Neut AP score

Answer to question 4.5

1. **Leuco-erythroblastic anaemia**
   Red and white cell precursors are present in the peripheral blood and the haemoglobin is low.

2 **Myelofibrosis**
   Although there are a number of conditions in which splenomegaly and a leuko-erythroblastic anaemia are associated, myelofibrosis is one condition in which both features are particularly common. Myelofibrosis is often asymptomatic but patients may complain of heaviness in the abdomen, due to the sheer bulk of the spleen. Other presenting features include tiredness, weight loss, pruritus, anorexia, gout, bone pain, jaundice and cramp.

   Causes of leuco-erythroblastic anaemia
   a. **Marrow infiltration** — due to
      carcinoma
      chronic leukaemia
      Myelofibrosis
      Multiple myeloma
      Malignant lymphoma
      Lipid storage disease
      Marble bone disease
      Tuberculosis
   b. **Severe hypoxia**
   c. **Marrow overactivity**

Question 4.6

A 28-year-old man is investigated for infertility.
Puberty was not delayed. The testicular volume was 10 ml.

Semen volume	2 ml
Sperm concentration	$5 \times 10^6/ml$
FSH	21.4 iu/l ↑
LH	17.2 iu/l ↑
Testosterone	3.6 nmol/l ↓
Prolactin	420 mu/l (N)

1. What is the diagnosis?
2. What other investigations should be performed?

Answer to question 4.6

1. Primary testicular failure

There is oligospermia (normal $\leq 20 \times 10^6$/ml) and elevation of LH and FSH, with a low serum testosterone. Impaired testosterone production by the Leydig cell stimulates gonadotrophin releasing hormone production resulting in elevated gonadotrophin levels by gonadal–hypothalmic negative feedback.

2. Chromosome analysis

The commonest cause of primary testicular failure is Klinefelter's syndrome (47 XXY karyotype). A buccal smear will be chromatin +ve with more than 20% of cells having Barr bodies.

Gynaecomastia may be present.

Question 4.7

A 2-month-old baby presents with fits:
Random glucose 6.4 mmol/l
Serum calcium 1.25 mmol/l
Serum phosphate 3.6 mmol/l
Alkaline phosphatase 320 iu/l
Urea 6.2 mmol/l

What is the most likely explanation?

Answer to question 4.7

Feeds with undiluted cow's milk

There is hypocalcaemia, and hyperphosphataemia with a normal blood sugar. The alkaline phosphatase is normal for a baby. The causes of hypocalcaemia in infancy are:

1. Neonatal hypoparathyroidism (in infants born to mothers with hyperparathyroidism)

2. Secondary to hyperphosphataemia:
   High phosphate feeds, e.g. cow's milk
   Renal failure

3. Calcium or vitamin D deficiency

Hypoparathyroidism is often accompanied by a slightly elevated serum phosphate but not of the order found in this case. This degree of hyperphosphataemia is only seen in high phosphate feeds or chronic renal failure. Significant renal failure is unlikely to be the cause as the urea is normal. Calcium or vitamin D deficiency would be associated with a normal or low rather than a high serum phosphate. In this case, as the phosphate is high, calcium phosphate may be precipitated and the ionised calcium concentration reduced. Alternatively the high phosphate may inhibit vitamin D activation.

Question 4.8

A 25-year-old Asian is admitted with headache and neck stiffness. He has been on no treatment.
CSF findings:
   Pressure 24 cm H_2O
   RBC 0
   WBC 275 $\times$ 10^6/l
      Lymphocytes 80%
      Monocytes 10%
      Neutrophils 10%
   Protein 0.8 mmol/l
   Glucose 1.8 mmol/l
   VDRL negative
Blood glucose 5.7 mmol/l

What is the diagnosis?

Answer to question 4.8

Tuberculous meningitis

There are four abnormal CSF findings:

1. CSF lymphocytosis — this occurs in:
   Tuberculous meningitis
   Viral meningitis
   Viral encephalomyelitis (especially mumps)
   Chronic meningococcal meningitis or
   partially treated bacterial meningitis
   Cerebral abscess
   Meningovascular syphilis
   CNS leukaemia, lymphoma
   Fungal meningitis
   Sarcoidosis

2. Lowering of CSF glucose (in the absence of hypoglycaemia). This is characteristic of bacterial meningitis but may also be rarely found in viral and fungal infections, sarcoidosis and malignancy.

3. Raised CSF protein. This can occur in any inflammatory lesion of the CNS.

4. Raised CSF pressure.

   Many of the above diseases could account for the CSF findings but tuberculosis is the most likely. It is particularly common in Asians.

Question 4.9

A 21-year-old man complains of haemoptysis and
lassitude:
Urea 16 mmol/l
Potassium 5.1 mmol/l
Serum albumin 21 g/l
Urinary protein 5g/24 h
Microscopy of urine: red cell casts + +

1. Give two possible diagnoses.
2. What three further investigations should be done?

Goodpastures

Answer to question 4.9

1. **Goodpasture's syndrome**
   Polyarteritis Nodosa (PAN)
   (A third possibility is Wegener's granulomatosis)
   The biochemical findings of renal failure combined with heavy proteinuria and red cell casts indicate an active glomerulonephritis. The only conditions giving acute glomerulonephritis with haemoptysis in this age group are Goodpasture's syndrome, polyarteritis nodosa, and Wegener's granulomatosis. Bronchial carcinoma with associated glomerulonephritis (usually membranous) occurs in later life. Goodpasture's syndrome has its peak incidence in the second and third decade, polyarteritis nodosa in the fifth and sixth decade. Both conditions are about three times commoner in men. Wegener's granulomatosis occurs in all age groups and is commoner in women.

2. a. **Chest X-ray** would show fluffy shadows of alveolar haemorrhages in Goodpasture's syndrome. Infiltrative shadows or pulmonary infarcts are seen in polyarteritis and Wegener's.
   b. **Anti-basement membrane antibodies** would be present in high titre in Goodpasture's and absent in Wegener's and polyarteritis.

   c. **Renal biopsy.** In Goodpasture's syndrome there is a diffuse proliferative glomerulonephritis with linear deposits of IgG and complement visible on immunofluorescence. In PAN medium and small arteries show the characteristic fibrinoid necrosis with a surrounding inflammatory reaction. In the glomerulus there may be focal or total necrosis with a surrounding inflammatory reaction. In Wegener's typical arterial wall granulomas are seen.

Question 4.10

A 50-year-old man with bruising:
Urea 15.0 mmol/l
Calcium 2.8 mmol/l
Alkaline phosphatase 84 iu/l
Total protein 85 g/l
Albumin 30 g/l
Haemoglobin 8.0 g/dl
MCV 100 fl
Platelets 15 × 10⁹/l
WBC 2.8 × 10⁹/l

1. What is the diagnosis?
2. Give two reasons for bruising.

Answer to question 4.10

1. **Myeloma**
   The correct diagnosis is indicated by the high globulin (55 g/l) obtained by subtracting the albumin from the total protein. The other features of myeloma in this patient are:
   a. Renal failure (the raised urea)
   b. Hypercalcaemia with the characteristically normal alkaline phosphatase
   c. A hypoplastic anaemia which could be caused by either the disease or its treatment

2. **Thrombocytopenia**
   Hyperviscosity syndrome
   Low levels of plasma clotting factors would be another satisfactory explanation.

Paper 5

Question 5.1

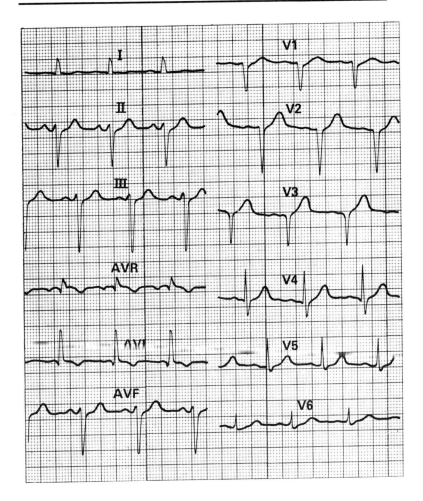

1. What abnormalities are present on the ECG?
2. What is the underlying diagnosis?

Answer to question 5.1

1. **The following abnormalities are present:**
   a. **Left axis deviation**
      The QRS axis is −60° consistent with marked left axis deviation. This is due to left anterior hemiblock.
   b. **Q waves in V3**
      There is definite pathological Q wave in V3 and a loss of R wave in V2 consistent with previous anterior infarction. The Q waves in AVR and AVL are not pathological being less than 0.2mV deep and 0.04 s long.
   c. **T wave inversion in AVL**
      The T wave axis is +90°. The angle between this and QRS axis (the QRS−T angle) is 150°. An angle of greater than 90° indicates significant myocardial disease.

2. **Previous anterior myocardial infarction** involving the anterior division of the left branch of the bundle of His (left anterior hemiblock).

Question 5.2

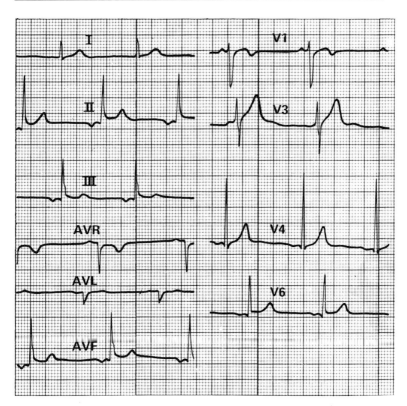

Routine pre-operative ECG on a 21-year-old man with no cardiac symptoms or signs.

1. What abnormalities (if any) are present?
2. Comment on the post-exercise ECGs.

After severe exercise: Ten minutes later:

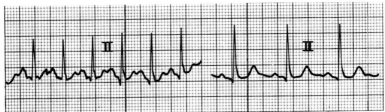

Answer to question 5.2

1. a. **Inverted P Waves** in leads II, III, AVF and V3–V6.
   b. **Short PR Interval — 0.12 s.**
   These two abnormalities suggest a resting nodal rhythm.
   Although Sokolows criteria for
   LVH ($SV_2 \times RV_5 > 35$ mm) are met, Romhilt and Estes
   criteria are not.

2. **He has reverted to sinus rhythm** with normal P waves
   and PR interval of 0.16 s.
   The resting nodal rhythm is an escape phenomenon seen
   in fit young subjects with high vagal tone causing sinus
   node suppression. Exercise causes an increase in sinus
   rate which then becomes the dominant rhythm. Atropine
   would have the same effect.

Question 5.3

A 21 stone lady aged 30 complains of continually
'dropping off' to sleep:
Chest X-ray normal
Peak flow 350 l/min
Haemoglobin 18.6 g/dl
WBC 6.3 × 10^9/l
Platelets 150 × 10^9/l

Arterial blood gases:
pO$_2$ 8 kPa
pCO$_2$ 7.5 kPa

1. What is the diagnosis?
2. Explain the raised haemoglobin.

Answer to question 5.3

1. Pickwickian syndrome

In this disease chronic respiratory failure is associated with gross obesity. The respiratory failure is due to hypoventilation. The cause of the hypoventilation is uncertain, but increased ventilatory effort due to obesity may be responsible. Some workers have suggested a hypothalamic lesion causing both the obesity and the hypoventilation. Primary lung disease is unlikely with a normal chest X-ray and near normal peak flow.

2. Secondary polycythaemia

This is due to the raised erythropoietin associated with prolonged hypoxaemia. Cor pulmonale is another feature.

Question 5.4

A 24-year-old homosexual man is seen in a venereology
clinic feeling unwell. He has no lymphadenopathy.
Bilirubin 35 μmol/l
Conjugated bilirubin 23 μmol/l
Alkaline phosphatase 110 iu/l
ALT 750 iu/l
AST 640 iu/l
VDRL negative

1. Give two possible diagnoses.
2. What four investigations would you perform?

Answer to question 5.4

1. a. **Infective hepatitis type B**
Type B may be sexually transmitted and is common in homosexuals as well as in drug addicts. The antigen has been isolated in semen.
   b. **Infectious mononucleosis**
Is spread by oral contact, is common in adolescents and frequently causes a hepatitis. A false positive VDRL may rarely occur. Rarely 2° syphilis may cause a diffuse hepatitis but a miliary granulomatous form is more common. Syphilis is more common in homosexuals. CMV and non A non B hepatitis may also be found in this group.

2. a. **HBsAg**
This will be found if the cause is type B hepatitis.
   b. **Fluorescent treponemal antibody test**
The VDRL test may occasionally give a biological false positive in all the above conditions. The FTA test is specific for treponemal infections. Killed treponemes are used as antigen and serum is added to the slide. The antibody is then made visible by the addition of fluorescence tagged anti-human globulin.
   c. **Paul-Bunnell**
If the cause is infectious mononucleosis, heterophile antibodies agglutinating sheep red cells adsorbed by ox red cells but not by guinea pig kidney will be present.
   d. **Urethral smear**
Any patient with a venereal disease, should be screened for gonorrhoea NSU and HIV serology.

Question 5.5

A 47-year-old female flower seller is admitted in late
October with dark urine, pyrexia and an early diastolic
murmur.
Haemoglobin 8.6 g/dl
Reticulocytes 15%
WBC 15.5 × 10⁹/l
   Neutrophils 75%
   Lymphocytes 23%
   Eosinophils 2%
Platelets 156 × 10⁹/l
Ham acid serum test: negative
Donath–Landsteiner test: positive
Fluorescent treponemal antibody (FTA): positive 1/160

1. What are the diagnoses?
2. Explain the heart murmur.

Answer to question 5.5

1. a. **Paroxysmal cold haemoglobinuria (PCH)**
      In paroxysmal cold haemoglobinuria haemolysis with haemoglobinuria is brought about by a cold haemolysin active against the patient's red cells. Acute haemolysis with anaemia, reticulocytosis, neutrophil leucocytosis, pyrexia and haemoglobinuria have been induced by the cold. In this case the time of year and occupation are obviously relevant. In the Donath–Landsteiner test clotted blood is cooled in iced water, allowing the cold haemolysin to unite with the red cells, and subsequently re-warmed when haemolysis occurs.

   b. **Syphilis**
      A positive FTA test is specific for active or inactive treponemal disease. Paroxysmal cold haemoglobinuria is said to occur in syphilis particularly in the congenital form. Other more common causes of PCH are mumps, measles and chicken pox.

2. **Syphilitic aortitis with aortic regurgitation**
   Infective endocarditis is not associated with cold haemolysins, a positive Donath–Landsteiner test or a positive FTA, though a false positive Wasserman reaction can occur.

Question 5.6

A 10-year-old boy has the following clotting screen:
Bleeding time 3 min 40 s
Whole blood clotting time 15 min, control 8 min
Prothrombin time 13 s control 12 s
Activated partial thromboplastin time: 80 s, control 12 s
Platelets $235 \times 10^9/l$

1. What is the most likely diagnosis?
2. What investigation would confirm this diagnosis?

Answer to question 5.6

1. Haemophilia a (factor VIII deficiency)

The bleeding time is normal but the whole blood clotting time is prolonged. A normal prothrombin time indicates functionally adequate levels of clotting factors II, V, VII and X. The prolonged partial thromboplastin time (PTT) indicates a functional deficiency of VIII, IX, XI, XII. The PTT may also be prolonged by circulating inhibitors of coagulation, and in this instance the addition of normal plasma will not correct the PTT.

Factor IX deficiency (Haemophilia B, Christmas disease) is clinically indistinguishable from haemophilia A but is much less common.

Factor XII (Hageman factor) deficiency is also very rare and not associated with clinical haemorrhage.

Factor XI deficiency resembles mild haemophilia and is very rare.

In Von Willebrand's disease the whole blood clotting time is usually normal and the bleeding time prolonged.

2. Factor VIII assay

The disease is severe when factor VIII levels are less than 1% of normal. The PTT may be normal in mild factor VIII and IX deficiency and cannot be used as a test to exclude haemophilia.

Question 5.7

A 35-year-old lady was complaining of a short history of
sore throat, dysphagia and a swelling in her neck. On
examination she had a slight tremor and tachycardia.
TSH 0.1 mu/l
Thyroxine 180 nmol/l
ESR 89 mm/h
Technetium^{99} thyroid uptake at 20 min 1.0%
Microsomal Ab −ve
Antithyroglobulin Ab −ve

1. What is the diagnosis?
2. What is the treatment?

Answer to question 5.7

1. **Acute thyroiditis (De Quervains)**
   This presents with a painful, enlarged thyroid often associated with symptoms of hyperthyroidism, because of the acute release of thyroxine and triiodothyronine. The thyroid gland is enlarged and may be very tender. In the early stages TSH secretion is suppressed but it may be differentiated from Graves disease by the very low radioiodine or technetium uptake. The ESR is frequently elevated. As the illness subsides the TSH will rise and isotope uptake will rise. It is thought to have a viral aetiology. A similar biochemical and thyroid scan occurs with thyrotoxicosis factitia.

2. Symptomatic treatment is necessary in most cases. If pain, fever and malaise are severe, a short course of corticosteroids will rapidly reduce the inflammation. 10% of cases are followed by permanent hypothyroidism.

Question 5.8

A 35-year-old housewife complains of generalised pruritus
for 3 years, and pale stools for 1 year.
Bilirubin 30 μmol/l
AST 45 iu/l
Albumin 32 g/l
Alkaline phosphatase 312 iu/l
Cholesterol 11.2 mmol/l

1. What is the likeliest diagnosis?
2. What is the cause of her pruritus?
3. Give one diagnostically useful blood test.

Answer to question 5.8

1. **Primary biliary cirrhosis (PBC)**
   Inflammation and fibrosis around intrahepatic bile ductules
   leads to intrahepatic cholestasis and retention of bile.
   This has two effects:
   a. Retention of biliary constituents, particularly bilirubin
   causing jaundice, and bile salts leading to pruritus. It
   also leads to hypercholesterolaemia.
   b. Malabsorption of fat causing steatorrhoea and
   deficiency of fat soluble vitamins.

2. **Retained bile salts**

3. **Antimitochondrial antibody titre** — this antibody is
   present in approximately 90% of patients with PBC but
   not in other types of cholestatic or obstructive jaundice.

Question 5.9

A 55-year-old male smoker presents with a three day
history of vomiting, weight loss of 12 lb over three months
and a history of recurrent abdominal pain.

Sodium	135 mmol/l
Potassium	3.1 mmol/l
Bicarbonate	40 mmol/l
Urea	12 mmol/l
Arterial [H]$^+$	32 nmol/l
Arterial pCO$_2$	6.0 KPa
Base excess	+ 18

1. What is the diagnosis?
2. What physical sign would you expect to find?
3. What is the metabolic abnormality?
4. What treatment would you institute?

Answer to question 5.9

1. **Pyloric stenosis**

2. **Gastric splash or visible peristalsis**

3. **Metabolic alkalosis**
   — there is a low hydrogen ion concentration (alkalosis)
   — the alkalosis is metabolic in origin because the plasma bicarbonate is elevated
   — the pCO_2 is at the upper end of the normal range
   — there is a base excess
   In respiratory alkalosis the pCO_2 is low secondary to hyperventilation and the plasma bicarbonate reduced.

4. Initial conservative management with nasogastric aspiration and fluid and electrolyte replacement. The diagnosis should be established by endoscopy to determine if the pyloric stenosis is a benign duodenal stricture secondary to duodenal ulceration or secondary to carcinoma of the pyloric antrum.

Question 5.10

A 35-year-old West Indian gives a 4-week history of
increasing headaches and progressive loss of vision. Her
blood pressure is found to be 210/135 mm/Hg
She has had no treatment.
Urea 35 mmol/l
Potassium 3.3 mmol/l
Sodium 130 mmol/l
Bicarbonate 10 mmol/l
Haemoglobin 9.6 g/dl

1. What is the diagnosis?
2. Why is her potassium low?

Answer to question 5.10

1. **Malignant (accelerated) hypertension with hypertensive encephalopathy**
   The high urea and low haemoglobin suggest chronic renal failure. The commonest causes are:
   a. Chronic glomerulonephritis
   b. Chronic pyelonephritis
   c. Obstructive uropathy
   d. Malignant hypertension
   e. Polycystic kidneys
   f. The collagenoses
   g. Amyloid disease
   h. Renovascular hypertension
   Malignant hypertension is suggested here by the race (it is relatively common in West Indians), the history of headaches and blindness due to encephalopathy and retinopathy, and the low potassium.

2. **Secondary hyperaldosteronism**
   The potassium is low because of secondary hyperaldosteronism resulting in the excretion of potassium in exchange for retained sodium, usually exceeding urinary sodium excretion. Hypokalaemia can occur even in the presence of moderately severe renal failure.
   Malignant hypertension causes narrowing of arterioles, particularly those supplying the juxtaglomerular apparatus. This results in low perfusion and a reflex hypersecretion of renin, which, via angiotensin causes excessive aldosterone release.

Paper 6

Question 6.1

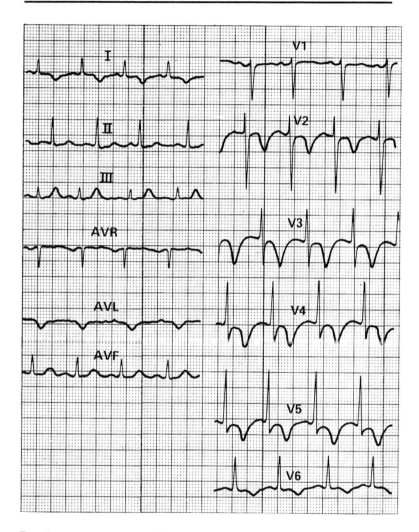

Routine pre-operative ECG on a 76-year-old lady with no cardiac symptoms or signs.

What is the diagnosis?

Answer to question 6.1

Antero-lateral subendocardial myocardial infarction
The ECG shows sinus arrhythmia. The only significant
abnormality is the deep T wave inversion in the antero-lateral
leads (I, AVL, V2–V6). T wave inversion of this magnitude
could also be caused by myocarditis but is usually more
widespread.

Question 6.2

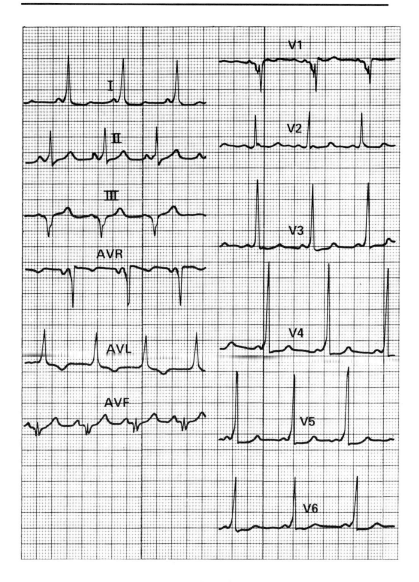

A 32-year-old woman with palpitations

1. What are the main abnormalities?
2. What is the diagnosis?

Answer to question 6.2

1. There are two abnormalities:
   a. **Shortest PR interval (0.08 s).**
   b. **A delta wave is present.** This is the slurring of the upstroke of the QRS complex which is best seen in leads V5 and V6.
2. **Type B Wolfe–Parkinson–White syndrome (WPW).**
   In this syndrome an abnormal bundle of conduction tissue bypasses the A-V node. Impulses passing down this bundle result in the early depolarisation (pre-excitation) of a part of the ventricle causing the delta wave. The rest of the QRS complex is normal as conduction via the A-V node and bundle of His occurs simultaneously.
   In type A WPW the aberrant bundle is situated on the left giving tall R waves in V1 and V2.
   In type B WPW the aberrant bundle is situated on the right giving a predominantly negative deflection in V1 as in this case.
   Both conditions may be associated with frequent attacks of paroxysmal supraventricular tachycardia, the cause of her palpitations. During an attack a circus movement develops. The impulse usually travels via the A-V node and bundle of His but 're-enters' the atria via the aberrant pathway, resulting in the loss of the delta wave. This is a rhythm strip of our patient during an acute attack, which demonstrates the change.

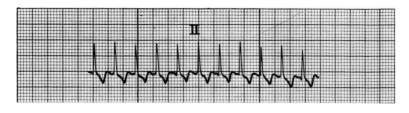

Question 6.3

A man aged 65 complains of dyspnoea.

	Before bronchodilator	After	Predicted
$FEV_{1.0}$ (l)	2.0	2.2	2.8
FVC (l)	5.2	5.3	4.0
PEFR (l/min)	345	360	540
Transfer factor TLCo	19.2		25.5
Permeability constant (KCo)	31		39

Answer to question 6.3

Emphysema

There is a greater reduction on FEV_1 than FVC with a reduced FEV_1/FVC ratio indicating airways obstruction, with little change following bronchodilator demonstrating limited reversibility. The pulmonary diffusion capacity is reduced due to a reduction in available gas exchange surface area hence the transfer factor is reduced. The permeability constant corrects for alterations in lung volume affecting the transfer factor.

Other causes of a low carbon monoxide transfer factor include:

Anaemia

Ventilation perfusion mismatch (e.g. pulmonary embolism)

Pulmonary fibrosis, oedema or infiltration

Reduced pulmonary diffusion area (e.g. post lung resection but in this case the KCo will be normal).

Question 6.4

A 30-year-old man develops severe left hypochondrial pain after a total hip replacement.
Pre-operative haemoglobin 12.0 g/dl
Film: 50% target cells

1. What is the diagnosis?
2. Explain his hypochondrial pain.
3. Why was his hip replaced?

Answer to question 6.4

1. Sickle-C disease

Sickle-C disease is characterised by a mild anaemia with a very high percentage of target cells.

Sickle cell anaemia is more severe (Hb < 9 g/dl) with target forms representing 4% at most of the total red cell population. In β-thalassaemia major target cells occur in large numbers, but the disease would not have allowed the patient to survive beyond childhood. Haemoglobin-C disease occurs in Negroes and causes a mild normochromic microcytic anaemia with 30–100% target cells. However, the complications described in this patient's history do not occur.

Sickle-thalassaemia tends to produce a moderate to severe anaemia which resembles homozygous sickle cell anaemia.

2. Splenic infarction

Sickling may be precipitated by hypoxia, e.g. flying in an unpressurised aircraft or anaesthesia. It may result in infarction of the spleen.

3. Avascular necrosis of the femoral head

Sickling may result in thrombosis in nutrient arteries. It also occurs in sickle cell disease and sickle-thalassaemia.

Causes of target cells:

Iron deficiency
Liver disease
Post-splenectomy
Haemoglobin-C
Sickle-cell anaemia
Thalassaemia

Question 6.5

A routine blood screen on a 25-year-old girl:
Haemoglobin 11.5 g/dl
MCV 62 fl
MCHC 28 g/dl
Reticulocytes 1%
Film: Anisocytosis
        Microcytosis
        Poikilocytosis
        Hypochromia
        Target cells
Serum iron 18 μmol/l

1. What is the diagnosis?
2. What test would confirm this?

Answer to question 6.5

1. Thalassaemia minor (thalassaemia trait)

There are two clues here:

a. The film appearances. These are similar to those of iron deficiency, since both disorders are due to a failure of haem synthesis.

b. The very low MCV. The differential diagnosis of thalassaemia minor is iron deficiency. In thalassaemia minor there is usually only a mild anaemia in conjunction with a very low MCV, whereas in iron deficiency both fall in proportion. The serum iron in this case is normal.

The other common forms of thalassaemia are:

(i) β-Thalassaemia major. There is a complete failure to synthesise chains and the patient relies on HbF and HbA_2 for haemoglobinisation. Presentation, even in its mildest form, occurs before the age of three with a moderately severe anaemia (Hb−6−10g/dl) jaundice, splenomegaly, retarded growth and malleolar ulcers. Characteristic facies and X-ray changes ('hair on end') are caused by widened marrow spaces. Gallstones and haemosiderosis are relatively late complications.

(ii) α-Thalassaemia major. This is incompatible with life, α-chains being necessary for the formation of fetal haemoglobin. It presents as hydrops fetalis.

(iii) α-Thalassaemia minor. The haemoglobin concentration is normal and the MCV only slightly reduced. The disease is asymptomatic.

2. Haemoglobin electrophoresis

This is the most useful diagnostic test. An increased percentage of haemoglobin A_2 is present in almost all cases of thalassaemia minor.

Question 6.6

A 65-year-old lady complains of being unable to comb her hair.
Haemoglobin 10.9 g/dl
MCV 98 fl
MCHC 34 g/dl
Sodium 128 mmol/l
Potassium 4.5 mmol/l
CPK 204 iu/l
ESR 30 mm/h
Lipid electrophoresis type IIa

1. What is the most likely diagnosis?
2. What two investigations would you perform to confirm the diagnosis?

Answer to question 6.6

1. **Primary hypothyroidism**
   She has four features of the disease
   a. Mild anaemia, macrocytosis and a mildly raised ESR.
   b. Hyponatraemia.
   c. Hyperlipidaemia. Friedrickson classification Type IIa may be secondary to hypothyroidism with an elevated cholesterol.
   d. Proximal myopathy. A proximal myopathy is a recognised feature of both hypo- and hyperthyroidism, although the elevated CPK in hypothyroidism probably originated from red blood cells.

2. a. Serum TSH which will be elevated in primary hypothyroidism and low in pituitary failure.
   b. Thyroid antibodies.

Question 6.7

A 35-year-old man with renal colic:
Urea 8.5 mmol/l
Sodium 142 mmol/l
Potassium 2.9 mmol/l
Bicarbonate 13 mmol/l
Calcium 2.4 mmol/l
Phosphate 1.0 mmol/l
Albumin 42 g/l

What is the diagnosis?

Answer to question 6.7

Renal tubular acidosis (RTA)

There is hypokalemic acidosis. In type 1 RTA the distal tubule fails to acidify the urine and sodium is exchanged for potassium instead of hydrogen ions. In type 2 RTA there is failure of hydrogen ion excretion in the proximal tubule. This may be associated with other features of proximal tubular dysfuncton, i.e. aminoacidaemia, renal glycosuria and phosphaturia-Fanconi syndrome.

Acidosis leads to increased calcium ionisation with hypercaluria leading to nephrocalcinosis, stones and osteomalacia, though total serum calcium is normal.

Causes of renal hypokalaemic alkalosis

a. Renal tubular acidosis
   Type 1 — Primary
          — Secondary — Autoimmune
                      — Nephrocalcinosis
                      — Drug induced
                      — Renal disease
   Type 2 — Multiple defects (Fanconi syndrome)
          — Primary
          — Secondary — Inborn errors of metabolism
                      — Hypocalcaemia
                      — Renal disease
                      — Drug induced
                      — Heavy metals
b. Acetazolamide
c. Partially treated diabetic ketoacidosis
d. Forced alkaline diuresis for salicylate overdose
e. Severe diarrhoea

NB: Hypokalaemia is usually associated with alkalosis.

Question 6.8

A manic-depressive of 30 complains of thirst.
She is apparently well controlled with lithium:
Serum lithium 0.95 mmol/l (therapeutic range
0.7–1.4 mmol/l)
After an 8 hour water deprivation test:
Urinary osmolality 300 mosm/kg
Plasma osmolality 295 mosm/kg
After 1 µg des-amino d-arginine vasopressin (DDAVP)
intramuscularly
Urinary osmolality 335 mosm/kg
Plasma osmolality 300 mosm/kg

What is the diagnosis?

Answer to question 6.8

Nephrogenic diabetes insipidus (DI) due to lithium
During a water deprivation test plasma osmolality should
not exceed 300 mosm/kg and urinary osmolality should
exceed 600 mosm/kg (i.e. twice the plasma osmolality).
Failure of this normal response indicates diabetes insipidus.
In psychogenic polydipsia furtive water ingestion during a
deprivation test may lead to failure of urine concentration but
plasma osmolality will remain normal or fall.
Failure of urinary concentration following DDAVP indicates
renal insensitivity to ADH; i.e. nephrogenic diabetes
insipidus. In cranial DI the abnormalities would be
corrected by DDAVP.
Nephrogenic DI may be caused by lithium even when the
serum levels are within the therapeutic range.

Question 6.9

Preliminary investigations of a 64-year-old man with a pyrexia of unknown origin:

Haemoglobin 18.2 g/dl

RBC 7200 $\times$ 10^9/l

WBC 7.5 $\times$ 10^9/l

 Neutrophils 65%

 Lymphocytes 32%

 Monocytes 3%

Platelets 330 $\times$ 10^9/l

MSU:

 RBC — 3000 $\times$ 10^6/l

 WBC — 0

 No other microscopic abnormality

 Culture — no growth

What is the diagnosis?

Answer to question 6.9

Hypernephroma

There is erythraemia (a raised red cell count) and blood in the urine. The combination is highly suggestive of hypernephroma, with secondary polycythaemia. Fever is a common feature of this condition. Other causes of erythraemia are:

1. Relative polycythaemia: e.g. stress, dehydration

2. True polycythaemia:
   a. Polycythaemia rubra vera
   b. Secondary polycythaemia:
      Hypoxia: eg. chronic bronchitis
      Inappropriate erythropoietin secretion:
      eg. liver carcinoma, renal tumours or cysts, cerebellar haemangioblastoma, phaeochromocytoma, uterine myomata

Question 6.10

A girl brings her 4-week-old infant to your clinic with an upper respiratory tract infection. You discover the girl has syphilis. The baby's serology is as follows:

VDRL positive, titre 1/16

FTA (Fluorescent treponemal antibody) positive, titre 1/320

FTA IgM positive, titre 1/80

1. Does the baby have syphilis?
2. Give the reason for your answer.

Answer to question 6.10

1. Yes

2. A positive IgM FTA in an infant indicates active disease. Only a few false positives are described in the literature. IgM does not cross the placenta and thus this antibody cannot reach the fetus by passive transfer. It must be synthesised by the infant. Although in healthy infants IgM synthesis does not begin until the age of 6 months, in congenital syphilis it begins sooner and the FTA IgM test can be positive at birth.

Paper 7

Question 7.1

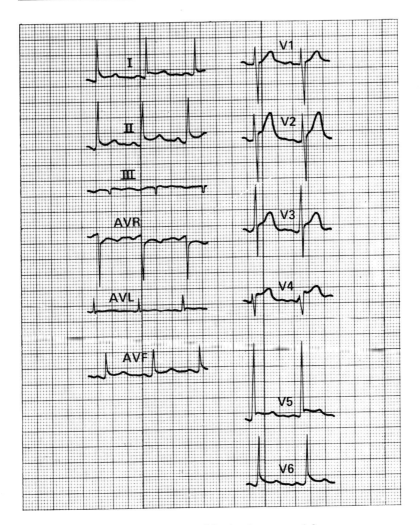

A 35-year-old man presents with tiredness and fever.

What is the diagnosis?

Answer to Question 7.1

Pericarditis
There is widespread ST elevation concave upwards. The extensive distribution of the changes and the absence of Q waves and T wave inversion make myocradial infarction unlikely.

The causes of pericarditis include:

Infections	— Viral — e.g. infectious mononucleosis, Coxsackie B
	Bacterial — e.g. staphylococcal, tuberculous
Drugs	— Hydrallazine
Inflammatory	— e.g. Rheumatic fever, SLE post cardiotomy and post myocardial infarction syndrome
Metabolic	— e.g. Uraemia, hypothyroidism
Trauma	
Malignancy	
Radiotherapy	

Question 7.2

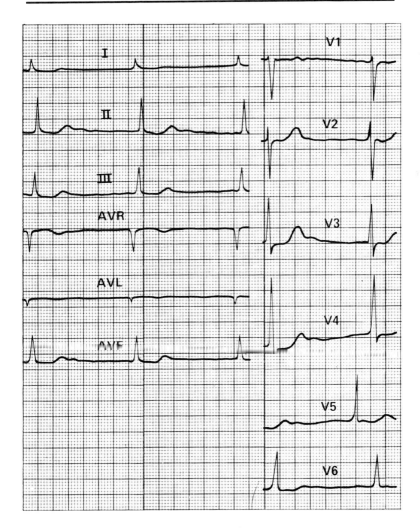

A 76-year-old man is brought into Casualty following an attack of unconsciousness. His wife has noticed a marked intellectual deterioration over the last six months.

1. Describe the main features of this ECG.
2. How would you treat this man?

Answer to question 7.2

1. **Atrial fibrillation with complete heart block**
   There is a profound bradycardia rate 41/min. The rhythm
   is regular but no P waves are seen. On careful
   examination fibrillation waves are visible in II and V1. The
   atrial rhythm is therefore **atrial fibrillation**.
   In the presence of atrial fibrillation a regular ventricular
   rhythm means that:
   a. the AV node is not conducting
   b. the ventricular pacemaker lies in the AV node or
      below.
      In this case, however, the normal QRS complex
      indicates that the pacemaker cannot be below the
      division of the bundle of His.

2. **Ventricular pacemaker**
   Cerebral perfusion will be improved and Stokes-Adams
   attacks will be prevented by pacing. A right ventricular
   pacemaker was inserted electively and ECG following this
   is shown below. It shows a pacing potential followed by
   a QRS complex with a left bundle block pattern.

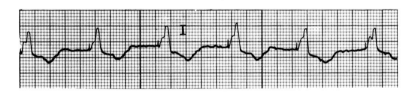

Question 7.3

A 50-year-old man is seen in the cardiac department
complaining of effort dyspnoea. A heart murmur is noted.
Cardiac catheter results:

Chamber	Pressure (mmHg)
Mean right atrium	3
Right ventricle	29/3
Pulmonary artery	28/14
Mean pulmonary artery wedge	18
Left ventricle	190/20
Aorta	110/80

Give two possible diagnoses.

Answer to question 7.3

1. **Aortic stenosis**
2. **Hypertrophic obstructive cardiomyopathy (HOCM)**
   There is a gradient of 80 mmHg across the region of the
   aortic valve. This could be due to stenosis of the value or
   to hypertrophy of the outflow tract — HOCM. These
   conditions can be distinguished by measurement of
   subvalvar pressure, left ventricular angiography and
   echocardiography. The left ventricular end diastolic
   pressure is raised. This may be due to left ventricular
   hypertrophy (thick non-compliant muscle) or to left
   ventricular failure.

Question 7.4

A 56-year-old cattle food manufacturer was admitted with weakness, lethargy and back pain. A CXR was normal. Renal calcification was seen on plain abdominal X-ray
Calcium 3.6 mmol/l
Phosphate 1.6 mmol/1
Urea 32 mmol/l
Creatinine 496 μmol/l
Albumin 36 g/l

1. What is the diagnosis?
2. What specific emergency treatment is indicated to reduce the hypercalcaemia?

Answer to question 7.4

1. Vitamin D intoxication

He has severe uraemia. The presence of hypercalcaemia and uraemia suggest the hypercalcaemia is causing the renal failure. The patient had been chronically ingesting vitamin D (which is added to cattle food) producing increased intestinal calcium absorption and bone resorption. Similar changes take place in phosphate transport. The prolonged increase in bone resorption produces rarefaction of bone and a subsequent crush fracture. The high calcium x phosphate product is responsible for metastatic calcification especially of renal tissue producing impaired renal function. The differential diagnosis includes sarcoidosis and malignancy. Hypercalcaemia in sarcoidosis is rarely seen without CXR changes. In the hypercalcaemia of malignancy the phosphate level may be variable but it would be unlikely to produce renal calcification.

2. Corticosteroids

The hypercalcaemia has produced severe renal impairment. Vitamin D metabolites may have a long half life, producing prolonged hypercalcaemia. In addition to general measures used to treat hypercalcaemia, corticosteroids are indicated and will induce a rapid reduction in the serum calcium.

Question 7.5

A 60-year-old West Indian man is admitted unconscious.

Blood glucose	72 mmol/l
Sodium	154 mmol/l
Potassium	4.9 mmol/l
Bicarbonate	22 mmol/l
Urea	19 mmol/l
Urine glucose	2%
Urine ketones (Ace test)	+

1. What is the diagnosis?
2. What four therapeutic measures would you institute?

Answer to question 7.5

1. **Hyperosmolar non ketotic coma**
   There is gross hyperglycaemia and dehydration is indicated by the high urea.
   The patient is not significantly acidotic because the plasma bicarbonate is only in the low normal range. The small quantity of urinary ketones does not indicate that ketoacidosis is present. Plasma ketone levels (assessed by testing undiluted plasma with acetest or ketosticks) will be greater than + + in ketoacidosis, and trace or small urinary ketones are common in any illness.
   The approximate plasma osmolarity is calculated as follows:
   $(2 \times Na^+) + (2 \times K^+) + $ blood glucose $+$ blood urea
   plasma osmalarity $= 408$ (NR 285–295)

2. a. Intravenous fluids — consider using 0.45% saline if sodium is greater than 150 mmol
   b. Intravenous insulin infusion — 2–6 unit/h
   c. Nasogastric tube
   d. Subcutaneous heparin
   The blood glucose and electrolytes should be carefully monitored and a precipitating cause identified.

   Types of coma in diabetes:
   Diabetic ketoacidosis
   Hyperosmolar coma
   Lactic acidosis (rare)
   Hypoglycaemia

Question 7.6

A previously fit 30-year-old woman complains of
tiredness:
Hb. 9.8 g/dl
MCV 94 fl
Film : Microcytes
        Macrocytes
        Target cells
        Howell-Jolly bodies
WBC 4.2 × 10⁹/1
        Right shift of neutrophils
Platelets 215 × 10⁹/1
Reticulocytes 0.8%
Urea 1.9 mmol/l
Electrolytes and liver function tests: normal

1. Explain the blood count findings.
2. What is the diagnosis?

Answer to question 7.6

1. The right shift of neutrophils and macrocytosis could be due to folate (or B_{12}) deficiency. Iron deficiency explains the microcytes and target cells. Howell–Jolly bodies, rarely seen in megaloblastic anaemia, are a common feature of splenectomy or splenic atrophy. Splenic atrophy is another cause of this patient's target cells.

2. Coeliac disease
The presence of a mixed deficiency anaemia and a low urea suggests malabsorption. There are also features of splenic atrophy which is a well-recognised complication of coeliac disease.

Question 7.7

A 23-year-old nurse complained of malaise and sore throat. Her GP gave her ampicillin which produced a rash. Investigations at that time:
Haemoglobin 13.6 g/dl
WBC 6.2 × 10⁹/1
Film: a few atypical lymphocytes

Three months later she developed purpura. Repeat blood test:
Haemoglobin 12.8 g/dl
WBC 6.5 × 10⁹/l
Platelets 15 × 10⁹/1

1. What was her first illness?
2. What was her second illness?

Answer to question 7.7

1. **Infectious mononucleosis**
   The main manifestations in this case are:
   a. Sore throat
   b. Malaise
   c. Rash. This is said to occur in up to 70% of patients with glandular fever who are given ampicillin.
   d. Atypical lymphocytes — though they may occur in other viral infections.
   Other manifestations include:
   Abdominal pain
   Hepatitis
   Splenomegaly
   Pericarditis and myocarditis
   Encephalitis, aseptic meningitis
   Peripheral neuritis
   Haemolytic anaemia

2. **Autoimmune thrombocytopenic purpura**
   This is a recognised complication of glandular fever. It is often associated with detectable anti-platelet antibodies.

Question 7.8

A 40-year-old woman with cataracts is referred from
psychiatric outpatients.
Calcium 1.50 mmol/l
Phosphate 1.75 mmol/l
Urea 5.0 mmol/l
Albumin 35 g/l

1. Give one possible diagnosis.
2. What two tests would you perform?

Answer to question 7.8

1. **Hypoparathyroidism**
   A low serum calcium associated with a high phosphate
   in the presence of normal renal function suggests
   either real or functional parathormone deficiency. In
   hypoparathyroidism (usually autoimmune or post-
   surgical), there is a genuine deficiency. In
   pseudohypoparathyroidism there is failure of the end
   organs to respond normally to parathormone.
   Although giving an identical biochemical picture
   pseudohypoparathyroidism presents in childhood.

2. **a.   Serum PTH.**
   This is low in hypoparathyroidism and high in
   pseudohypoparathyroidism.
   b.   The Ellsworth-Howard test
   Parathormone is administered. In true hypoparathyroidism
   there is a marked rise in the urinary phosphate excretion
   and a twenty-fold increase in urinary cyclic AMP. In
   pseudohypoparathyroidism these changes do not occur.

Question 7.9

A 53-year-old woman suddenly starts bruising easily. She brings some tablets with her, which she has been taking for 2 years. It is not clear whether these were prescribed or bought from her chemist.

Haemoglobin 8.0 g/dl
MCV 82 fl
WBC 2.1 × 10^9/1
   Neutrophils 25%
   Lymphocytes 75%
Platelets 30 × 10^9/1
   Thyroxine 15 nmol/l
TSH 25 mU/l

What were the tablets?

Answer to question 7.9

There are two possibilities:

1. **Antithyroid drugs, e.g. carbimazole, propylthiouracil.**
2. **Phenylbutazone and related drugs.**
   She has a pancytopenia which is commonly induced by
   phenylbutazone and antithyroid drugs, and usually
   appears suddenly. Hypothyroidism is another rare
   complication of phenylbutazone therapy. Antithyroid
   drugs will produce hypothyroidism if used in excessive
   dosage, or for prolonged periods.

   ### Some complications of phenylbutazone therapy
   a. Gastrointestinal haemorrhages
   b. Interference with oral anticoagulants
   c. Fluid retention
   d. Skin rashes, e.g. erythema multiforme
   e. Nausea
   f. Pancytopenia, agranulocytosis etc.
   g. Hypothyroidism

Question 7.10

A 40-year-old man with a cough and weakness in his legs
has the following CSF findings:
Pressure 11 cm H_2O
Protein 4.75 g/l
Sugar 4.0 mmol/l
Cells: RBC — none seen
         WBC — 4 lymphocyte/ml
Blood glucose 6.0 mmol/l

List your differential diagnosis.

Answer to question 7.10

1. Guillain-Barré syndrome
The raised CSF protein is secondary to an inflammatory exudate from nerve roots. It commonly presents with weakness in the legs, with arm and respiratory involvement occurring later (Landry's ascending paralysis). The cough could be due to an antecedent respiratory infection.

2. Froin's syndrome
Features of this CSF are typical of Froin's syndrome with a normal pressure and grossly elevated protein content. Froin's syndrome is characterised by spinal cord compression leading to impaired venous drainage and oedema of the cord. His cough could be due to a bronchial carcinoma, with a deposit in the spinal cord.

3. Carcinomatous neuropathy
When nerve roots are involved in this condition, the CSF protein will be high. It generally presents as a mixed sensory and motor neuropathy.

Causes of raised CSF protein above 2/gl
Guillain-Barré syndrome
Froin's syndrome
Carcinomatous neuropathy
Neurofibromata including acoustic neuroma
Meningitis   —   acute bacterial
                 tuberculous
                 fungal

Paper 8

Question 8.1

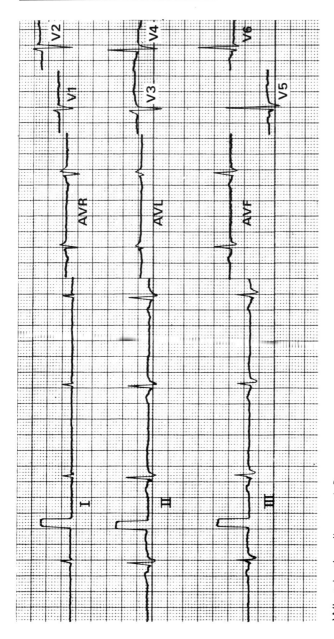

What is the diagnosis?

Answer to question 8.1

Hypothyroidism

The following abnormalities point to the correct diagnosis:

1. Sinus bradycardia — rate 54/min.

2. Lowering of QRS voltage. This is usually more marked than in this ECG. It may be caused by myxoedematous changes in the myocardium, pericardial effusion, increased skin electrical resistance or by a combination of these factors.

3. Flattened T waves in all leads.
   Lengthening of the Q–T interval may also be seen in hypothyroidism but is not present on this ECG. All changes are reversed by thyroxine.

Question 8.2

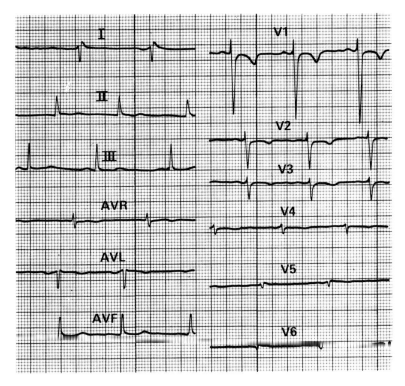

A 32-year-old man is referred to the cardiac clinic with an ECG taken at an insurance examination.

1. What is the diagnosis?
2. What abnormalities may be associated with this condition?

Answer to question 8.2

1. **Dextrocardia**
   The following abnormalities are present:
   a. **Right axis deviation (axis greater than +90°)**
      The negative QRS complex in lead I with the isoelectric QRS in AVF means that the axis is +120°. The causes of right axis deviation are:
   (i) Right ventricular hypertrophy, e.g. mitral stenosis, cor pulmonale.
   (ii) Tall, asthenic subjects.   (iii) Left posterior hemiblock.
   (iv) Secundum atrial septal defect.   (v) Dextrocardia.
   b. **Progessive loss of QRS voltage in the chest leads.** This is only seen in dextrocardia and occurs as the exploring electrode moves further from the heart. When right sided V leads are recorded QRS progression is normal.

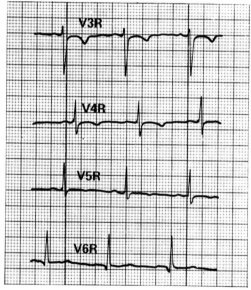

2. a. **Situs inversus.** A complete mirror image with transposition of all viscera. Apart from their position the viscera (including the heart) are all normal.
   b. **Kartagener's syndrome.** Bronchiectasis, sinusitis, dextrocardia, situs inversus.
   c. **Partial transposition of the viscera.** This is often associated with other serious cardiac abnormalities.

Question 8.3

A 50-year-old woman with nausea and anorexia:
Calcium 1.63 mmol/l
Phosphate 2.50 mmol/l
Urate 0.88 mmol/l
Alkaline phosphatase 180 iu
Albumin 32 g/l

1. What is the diagnosis?

Answer to question 8.3

Chronic renal failure

A high urate and phosphate are secondary to renal failure. There is hypocalcaemia secondary to phosphate retention and vitamin D resistance, which may contribute to uraemic bone disease. The plasma alkaline phosphatase is commonly raised in renal failure but is not always due to increases in the bone derived fraction. The high calcium/phosphate product may lead to metastatic calcification.

Hypoalbuminemia lowers total calcium but ionised calcium levels remain normal.

Question 8.4

A 56-year-old woman with rheumatoid arthritis has
postural faints. Blood pressure 110/60 lying, 90/50
standing. She has no oedema. Her current treatment is
indomethacin 25 mg t.d.s.
Urea 8.0 mmol/l
Sodium 129 mmol/l
Potassium 4.9 mmol/l
Urinary sodium 74 mmol/24 h after 18 h fluid
deprivation
Synacthen test: 9 am Cortisol 331 nmol/l
$\frac{1}{2}$ h after synacthen 628 nmol/l
1 h after synacthen 600 nmol/l
Supine plasma aldosterone 1040 pmol/l (NR: 100-600)

1. What is the underlying metabolic abnormality?
2. Name two possible causes related to her rheumatoid
   arthritis.

Answer to question 8.4

1. **Salt losing nephritis**
   The patient is salt depleted. The high urinary sodium
   following water deprivation (>60 mmol/24 h) points to
   the loss being in the urine. This suggests a renal lesion as
   she is not on diuretics. The normal cortisol response
   excludes Addison's disease, and with the elevated
   aldosterone level, reflects the low plasma volume
   associated with salt depletion.

2. **a. Analgesic nephropathy**
   b. Amyloid disease
   Although this usually presents as the nephrotic
   syndrome, salt losing nephritis may occur if the amyloid is
   predominantly deposited in the tubules.
   Other causes of salt losing nephritis are those where the
   disease has its major effect on the tubles. They include:
   Chronic pyelonephritis
   Obstructive uropathy
   Polycystic disease
   Nephrocalcinosis
   Hyperuricaemia
   Myeloma
   Wilson's Disease
   Heavy metal poisons
   Recovery phase of acute tubular necrosis
   Cystic disease of the medulla

Question 8.5

A 55-year-old woman with a rash and muscle weakness:
Sodium 141 mmol/l
Potassium 4.2 mmol/l
Calcium 2.45 mmol/l
AST 115 iu/l
Creatinine phosphokinase (CPK) 750 iu/l

1. What is the diagnosis?
2. What diseases are associated with this disorder?

Answer to question 8.5

1. **Dermatomyositis**
   The patient has a rash and abnormal enzymes, probably originating from muscle. This is suggestive of dermatomyositis. Aldolase is another muscle enzyme that will be raised in this condition.

2. It is often associated with autoimmune connective tissue diseases such as scleroderma or SLE. It may be a manifestation of internal malignancy, particularly in the older age group.

   Causes of a raised CPK:
   Myocardial infarction
   Muscle injury (including intra-muscular injection)
   Muscular dystrophies
   Myxoedema
   Severe physical exertion
   Alcoholism

Question 8.6

Following an upper respiratory infection a medical student
is noticed to be icteric:
Total bilirubin 52 µmol/l
AST 21 iu/l
Alkaline phosphatase 42 iu/l
Urine: bilirubin — negative
        urobilinogen — positive
Haemoglobin 15.2 g/dl
Reticulocytes 0.7%

1. What is the diagnosis?
2. What treatment is available for the icterus?

Answer to question 8.6

1. **Gilbert's disease**
   In the presence of an elevated plasma bilirubin the
   absence of bilirubin in the urine suggests that the excess
   of circulating bilirubin is unconjugated (non water soluble).
   There is no evidence of haemolysis, hepatic disease or
   biliary disease. Gilbert's disease is a harmless congenital
   abnormality in which there is underactivity of bilirubin
   UDP–glucuronyl transferase. The clinical jaundice is
   intermittent and usually only detectable during an
   intercurrent illness, although the serum bilirubin may also
   be elevated by fasting. The distinction from haemolysis
   may sometimes be difficult and further investigation may
   be necessary. Some patients may have a decreased red
   cell survival.

2. **Enzyme inducing agents** such as phenobarbitone may
   be used in those with noticeable jaundice between
   attacks to produce a cosmetic improvement.

Question 8.7

A 6-year-old boy from Glasgow is admitted with
abdominal pain and constipation. There are no skin lesions.
Hb. 9.1 g/dl
MCV 86 fl
Urea 10.7 mmol/l
Urine: δ-amino-laevulinic acid present
   24-hour urinary coproporphyrin 0.5 μmol/24 h
   (NR:< 0.25)

1. What is the diagnosis?
2. List three complications that can occur.

Answer to question 8.7

1. Lead poisoning

There is a normocytic anaemia. Punctuate basophilia due to precipitated RNA in the red cell is often present, but is not specific for lead poisoning. It also occurs in pernicious anaemia, leukaemias and many of the haemoglobinopathies. The absence of skin lesions excludes congenital erythropoetic porphyria, the only variant in which anaemia is a feature. The raised urea is evidence of the nephro-toxicity of lead. Lead inhibits the formation of δ-amino-laevulinic acid (δ-ALA), its conversion to porphobilinogen and the incorporation of iron into protoporphyrin to form haem. This leads to the accumulation of δ-ALA and coproporphyrin III in the blood and their excretion in the urine. Failure of incorporation of iron may lead to a sideroblastic anaemia. Lead poisoning is relatively common in Glasgow where exposure to lead in water (lead pipes), paint and car exhaust fumes is frequent.

2. Anaemia
   Nephrotoxicity
   Encephalopathy
   Peripheral neuropathy
   are all complications of lead poisoning.

Question 8.8

A lady of 65 complains of feeling tired. She has had three
attacks of bronchitis in the last six months:
Hb. 6.7 g/dl
MCV 106 fl
Reticulocytes 25%
Film: polychromasia
        spherocytosis
WBC 115 $\times$ 10^9/l
    neutrophils 10%
    lymphocytes 90%
Platelets 95 $\times$ 10^9/l
Direct Coombs' test: positive

1. What are the diagnoses?
2. Name two therapeutic measures you would employ.

Answer to question 8.8

1. a. **Autoimmune haemolytic anaemia**
      There is a profound anaemia with a high reticulocyte
      count consistent with haemolysis or haemorrhage. The
      spherocytosis suggests haemolysis and the positive
      Coombs' test demonstrates that the process is
      autoimmune. The polychromasia and macrocytosis
      reflects the high reticulocyte count.
   b. **Chronic lymphatic leukaemia (CLL)**
      The very high lymphocyte count is diagnostic of CLL.
      Autoimmune haemolytic anaemia occurs in 10–25%.

2. a. **Corticosteroids** usually rapidly control the haemolysis
      with a rise in haemoglobin and a falling reticulocyte
      count. A starting dose of 40–60 mg prednisolone a
      day is usual, the dose being reduced as the patient
      goes into remission. Corticosteroids will also lower the
      lymphocyte count and the thrombocytopenia of CLL
      may respond to steroids.
   b. **Chlorambucil** — high dose intermittent treatment
      with this drug should aim at reducing the white blood
      count to around 15 $\times$ 10^9/l

Indications for treatment:
   1. Impaired marrow function, ie. anaemia, neutropenia or
      thrombocytopenia.
   2. Autoimmune haemolytic anaemia.
   3. Marked enlargement or lymph nodes or spleen.
A high white count alone is not an indication for treatment.
Observation is all that is required.

Question 8.9

An Irish labourer presents with weight loss and diarrhoea:
Haemoglobin 12.0 g/dl
MCV 98 fl
MCHC 35 g/dl
WBC 4.5 $\times$ 10^9/l
Faecal fat 82 mmol/24 h on 100 g fat diet
Xylose test 20% of dose excreted in 2 h
Fasting glucose 9.5 mmol/l
Alkaline phosphatase 62 iu/l

1. What is the diagnosis?
2. What investigations would confirm the diagnosis?

Answer to question 8.9

1. Chronic pancreatitis

There is evidence of malabsorption and mild diabetes. The malabsoprtion is demonstrated by steatorrhoea (normal faecal fats less than 18 mmol/24 h). The raised MCV could be due to associated chronic alcoholism with or without folate deficiency. The main types of malabsorption are:

a. Intestinal. The normal xylose absorption is against this.

b. Biliary obstruction. This would be associated with a high alkaline phosphatase.

c. Pancreatic. The associated diabetes makes this the most likely diagnosis.

2. a. **Plain abdominal X-ray** — to show pancreatic calcification.

b. **Lundt test meal** — impaired pancreatic function may be demonstrated by reduced concentration of bicarbonate and pancreatic enzymes in the aspirate.

c. **Endoscopic retrograde cholangiopancreatography (ERCP)** will show tortuosity and dilatation, sometimes with stricture formation of the main pancreatic duct and loss of the fine feathery pattern of the side ductules.

The following investigations, though important in assessment, are less helpful in diagnosis:

a. Serum folate.

b. Serum iron. This is sometimes reduced in intestinal, but not usually in pancreatic, malabsorption.

c. Serum calcium. ⎱ Both may be abnormal due
d. Prothrombin time. ⎰ to malabsorption of fat soluble vitamins D and K.

e. Liver function tests. Raised liver enzymes, particularly the γ-glutamyl transpeptidase, may result from coexistent alcoholic liver disease.

f. Serum albumin.

Serum amylase is not indicated as it is normal in chronic pancreatitis except during acute exacerbations. The fasting blood glucose is well above normal and a glucose tolerance test is thus unnecessary to diagnose diabetes.

Question 8.10

Investigations of a thirsty baby boy:
Plasma osmolality 310 mosm/kg
Urinary osmolality 210 mosm/kg
Antidiuretic hormone level 9.5 pmol/l (NR: 0.9–4.6 pmol/l)

What is the diagnosis?

Answer to question 8.10

Nephrogenic diabetes insipidus

Dilute urine in the presence of concentrated plasma results from failure of ADH-dependent water reabsorption in the kidney, i.e. diabetes insipidus (DI). The high ADH indicates that this baby's renal tubules are unresponsive to ADH, signifying nephrogenic rather than pituitary DI. The condition is inherited as a sex-linked recessive.

Acquired nephrogenic DI may be the result of renal tubular failure from any cause, for example: uric acid nephropathy, hypercalcaemia, hypokalaemia, lithium.

Paper 9

Question 9.1

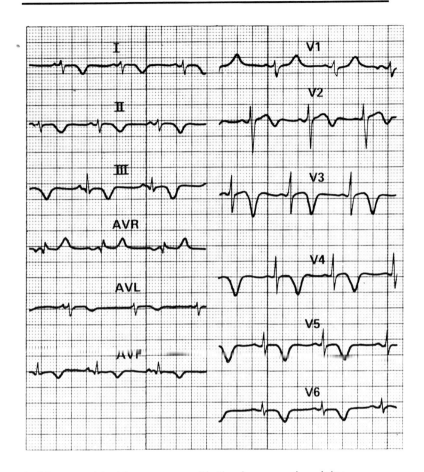

A 23-year-old girl presents with tiredness and malaise.

What is the diagnosis?

Answer to question 9.1

Myocarditis

There is widespread and deep T wave inversion of a degree which can only occur in myocarditis or subendocardial infarction. In this case the latter is unlikely in view of the age of the patient and the extent of the T wave changes.

Although a cardiomyopathy may give this degree of T wave inversion, this is not usual and the history suggests a viral infection. The distinction between myocarditis and a cardiomyopathy is somewhat artificial but myocarditis usually implies an infective aetiology.

The main causes are:

a. Viruses   Coxsackie
influenza
infectious mononucleosis
b. Bacterial: diphtheria
rheumatic fever
c. Parasitic: Chagas disease
toxoplasmosis

Question 9.2

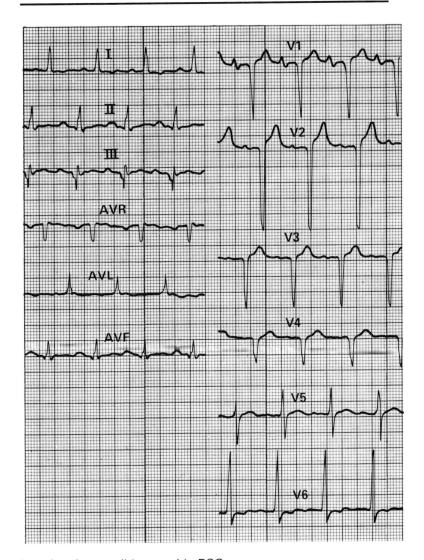

List the abnormalities on this ECG.

Answer to question 9.2

1. **Left atrial hypertrophy**
   This is best seen in V1 where there is a biphasic P wave. The negative component of this represents prolonged left atrial depolarisation. It fulfils the criteria of left atrial hypertrophy by exceeding 1 mm depth and 0.04 s in duration.

2. **First degree heart block**
   The PR interval is 0.23 s. The upper limit of normal is generally taken as 0.22 s.

3. **Left ventricular hypertrophy**
   T wave inversion in the lateral chest leads (I, AVL and V6) sometimes with ST depression is a common feature of left ventricular hypertrophy. This is often referred to as 'strain' pattern.

4. **Q Waves in III, V1 to V4**
   Suggesting previous anterior and inferior infarction. The small Q wave in AVF is not strictly speaking pathological as it is less than 0.04 s wide and less than 2 mm deep.

Question 9.3

A 60-year-old man has the following blood count:
Haemoglobin 19.6 g/dl
RBC 8200 $\times$ 10^9/l
PCV 65%
WBC 21 $\times$ 10^9/l
    Neutrophils 85%
    Lymphocytes 15%
Platelets 800 $\times$ 10^9/l
ESR 1 mm/hr
Leucocyte alkaline phosphatase (LAP) score 85/100
neutrophils (NR: 20–70)

He is given some treatment, recovers and is lost to follow
up. He is seen again 9 years later and his blood count is
then:
Haemoglobin 8.5 g/dl
RBC 2800 $\times$ 10^9/l
WBC 13 $\times$ 10^9/l
    Myeloblasts 90%
    Neutrophils 2%
    Polymorphs 2%
    Lymphocytes 6%
Platelets 45 $\times$ 10^9/l

1. What was the original diagnosis?
2. What was the therapy?
3. What is the current diagnosis?
4. List three other complications of the first diagnosis.

Answer to question 9.3

1. **Polycythaemia rubra vera (PRV)**

   There is an increase in all blood cellular constituents. In secondary polycythaemia only the red cell count is raised. In PRV about 75% have a raised white count and 66% have a thrombocythaemia. The LAP score is usually raised in PRV and normal in secondary polycythaemia, unless there is infection.

2. **P^{32}**

   3–7 millicuries intravenously is usually sufficient to achieve remission with a fall of all indices to normal. Remissions may last from a few months to several years. In this case preliminary venesection would also have been necessary as the PCV was more than 55%. Chlorambucil is no longer used but other alkylating agents or hydroxyurea may be used as myelosuppressive therapy.

3. **Acute myeloid leukaemia**

   Circulating myeloblasts in these numbers are pathognomonic of this disease. Acute leukaemia is a late complication of PRV usually occurring after about 10 years. It is possibly slightly commoner in patients who have had P^{32}, but the improved life expectancy (from about 7 years untreated to about 13 years treated) justifies its use. It may occur spontaneously as a late complication of PRV. Chlorambucil is no longer used as a treatment because trials have shown an increased incidence of leukaemic transformation.

4. **Complications of PRV:**

   Thrombosis:
      myocardial infarction
      pulmonary infarction
      arterial thrombosis in any site
   Haemorrhage:
      epistaxis
      post traumatic and surgical
      spontaneous — especially GI cutaneous and cerebral
   Hypertension
   Hyperuricaemia and gout
   Peptic ulceration
   Myelosclerosis
   Leukaemic transformation

Question 9.4

A man being treated for Crohn's disease presents with
tetany.
Calcium 2.10 mmol/l
Phosphate 0.85 mmol/l
Albumin 28 g/l
Potassium 3.7 mmol/l
Bicarbonate 25 mmol/l
PO_2 12.6 kPa
PCO_2 5.9 kPa

What is the probable cause of this man's tetany?

Answer to question 9.4

Hypomagnesaemia

Magnesium deficiency causes symptoms similar to hypocalcaemia. The serum calcium is appropriate for the low plasma albumin. Hyperventilation may lower plasma ionised calcium but in this case ventilation is normal as manifested by a normal PCO_2.

Causes of Hypomagnesaemia

a. Severe prolonged diarrhoea, including fistula, ileostomy, etc.
b. Malabsorption
c. Prolonged parenteral nutrition
d. Diuretic therapy
e. $1°$ + $2°$ Hyperaldosteronism
f. Hypoparathyroidism
g. Diabetic coma
h. Chronic alcoholism and cirrhosis
i. Cisplatinum chemotherapy

Question 9.5

An elderly lady is referred to the thyroid clinic by her
general practitioner who has been treating her for
hypothyroidism for two years.
Thyroxine 104 nmol/l
TSH 16 mu/l
Free T4 24 pmol/l (NR 8.8–23)

Give possible explanations.

Answer to question 9.5

1. **Non-compliance**
   These are discrepant results. The elevated TSH is
   suggestive of hypothyroidism but serum thyroxine levels
   are normal and free T4 levels slightly elevated. This is
   characteristic of intermittent compliance with therapy.
   The serum thyroxine rises rapidly with treatment but
   prolonged compliance may be needed to achieve
   adequate 'tissue levels' of thyroxine and suppress TSH.
   This patient had only begin to comply with therapy
   recently because of an imminent outpatient appointment.

2. A similar biochemical picture would be found in an
   individual who had recently commenced treatment for the
   first time.

Question 9.6

A 65-year-old lady with previously normal renal function becomes oliguric following abdominal surgery.

Urea	19.0mmol/l
Sodium	130mmol/l
Potassium	5.9mmol/l
Glucose	6.4mmol/l
Creatinine	120µmol/l
Urine osmolality	504mosm/Kg

1. Why is she oliguric?
2. What treatment does she need?

Answer to question 9.6

1. Pre renal failure (dehydration)

A raised plasma urea in a patient with previously normal renal function is likely to be due to dehydration or acute renal failure.

The high plasma urea/creatinine ratio is suggestive of dehydration. This is confirmed by the urine plasma osmolality ratio being greater than 1.5. To calculate the plasma osmolarity use the formula

2Na + 2K + urea + glucose. In pre-renal failure tubular function is normal producing a concentrated urine with a high urea and osmolality and with a low sodium. In acute tubular necrosis tubular function is impaired. Pre renal uraemia can be distinguished from renal failure by other urinary measurements.

	Pre Renal	Renal
Urine sodium (mmol/l)	<20	>40
Urine osmolality (mOsm/Kg)	>500	<400
Urine/plasma urea ratio	>10	<10

These tests cannot be interpreted unless oliguria is present and diuretics have not been used.

2. Intravenous normal saline

Question 9.7

A 20-year-old girl with secondary amenorrhoea presents to rheumatology outpatients with painful wrists. She has slight jaundice and hepatosplenomegaly. She is on no therapy.

Haemoglobin 13.2 g/dl
ESR 32 mm/hr
ALT 225 iu/l
AST 182 iu/l
Bilirubin 40 μmol/l
Alkaline phosphatase 80 iu/l
Anti-nuclear factor (ANF) positive 1/128
DNA binding 12 U (NR: ≤25)
Smooth muscle antibodies positive
LE cells negative

What is the diagnosis?

Answer to question 9.7

Chronic active hepatitis (CAH)

The clinical features and antibody screen are typical of this disease. The liver function tests show a hepatocellular jaundice.

The incidence of positive antibodies in CAH is:

ANF 25–75%

Raised DNA binding 5–20% (the exact incidence has not been determined)

Smooth muscle antibodies 50–80%

LE cells 15%

The causes of hepatocellular jaundice are:

1. Infections — eg. 'infectious hepatitis' types A or B, infectious mononucleosis, cytomegalovirus, toxoplasmosis.

2. Toxic, e.g. alcohol, paracetamol, MAOIs.

3. Drug allergies, e.g. methyldopa

4. Genetic, e.g. Wilson's disease, galactosaemia.

Hepatitis in SLE is rare and is likely to be associated with positive LE cells and a raised DNA binding.

Primary biliary cirrhosis (PBC) may be associated with positive smooth muscle antibodies (30%) though anti-mitochondrial antibodies are more usual (90%). In addition the patient with PBC usually falls into an older age group and the jaundice is cholestatic rather than hepatocellular.

Question 9.8

A 35-year-old man complains of weight loss and
abdominal distention. Three years ago he was treated
successfully for an itchy vesicular rash on his buttocks.
Haemoglobin 8.3 g/dl
MCHC 29 g/dl
MCV 96 fl

Film: macrocytosis+
    : microcytosis+
    : anisocytosis++
    : poikilocytosis+

1. What is the diagnosis?
2. What investigations would confirm the diagnosis?
3. What was the rash?

Answer to question 9.8

1. Coeliac disease

He has a mixed macrocytic and microcytic anaemia suggesting both iron and folate (possibly B_{12}) deficiency. This is a characteristic feature of coeliac disease being due to upper intestinal malabsorption. Crohn's disease, small bowel lymphoma, Whipple's disease, giardiasis and partial gastrectomy could give a similar haematological picture but in this case the itchy rash should give a clue to the correct diagnosis. Remember that malabsorption due to pancreatic disease does not usually cause iron deficiency.

2. Jejunal biopsy

A jejunal biopsy via a Crosby capsule or a duodenal biopsy via a duodenoscope would show flattening of the mucosal villi, and infiltration of the lamina propria with inflammatory cells. The abnormalities reverse when the patient is treated with a gluten free diet for a year.
Some authorities claim it is necessary to do a third biopsy after a rechallenge with gluten to be absolutely certain of the diagnosis especially in young children. Cow's milk sensitivity and infectious enteritis may induce similar mucosal lesions which can spontaneously improve whilst on a gluten free diet.

3. Dermatitis herpetiformis

This itchy vesicular rash is strongly associated with coeliac disease. It is claimed that dermatitis herpetiformis may often respond to a gluten free diet alone though dapsone is the more conventional treatment. Both dermatitis herpetiformis and coeliac disease are strongly correlated with the HLA B8 and DRW3 antigen.

Question 9.9

A 19-year-old secretary is admitted in a restless and confused state. She is pale, sweaty, tachypnoeic and oliguric:

Arterial blood gases:

PO_2 12.6 kPa

PCO_2 3.2 kPa

pH 7.08

Blood glucose 8.2 mmol/l

Urine analysis: glucose $\frac{1}{4}$% ketones $+$

1. What is the diagnosis?
2. What three other investigations would you perform?

Answer to question 9.9

1. She has a severe metabolic acidosis causing hyperventilation reflected in the low PCO_2 and raised PO_2. The causes of severe metabolic acidosis are:
a. Salicylate poisoning
b. Diabetic ketoacidosis
c. Renal failure
d. Lactic acidosis (very unusual in this age group).
Other causes of metabolic acidosis are usually less severe. They include:
e. Renal tubular acidosis
f. Diarrhoea
g. Acetazolamide therapy
h. Ureterocolic anastomosis
The most likely diagnosis is salicylate poisoning when buffering mechanisms have been overcome giving a severe metabolic acidosis. Mild hyperglycaemia is common as is moderate ketonuria. Salicylate in the urine may give a false positive reaction with ketosticks.

2. a. Salicylate level
   b. Urea and electrolytes
   c. Clotting studies

Question 9.10

A 68-year-old woman complains of left loin pain. She had
an abdominal operation 5 years ago:
Urea 12.5 mmol/l
Sodium 143 mmol/l
Potassium 3.1 mmol/l
Bicarbonate 15 mmol/l
Chloride 114 mmol/l

1. What operation has been performed?
2. What treatment does she require?

Answer to question 9.10

1.   **Ureteroenterostomy**
      The features are hypokalaemic hyperchloraemic
      acidosis and mild uraemia. The bowel, unlike the
      bladder is capable of active transport of ions. Chloride
      is reabsorbed in exchange for bicarbonate producing
      the hyperchloraemic acidosis. Urea is split by urease-
      containing bowel coliforms releasing ammonia. This is
      reabsorbed and urea is reconstituted in the liver,
      creating an entero-hepatic circulation of urea.
      Transplantation of the ureters into the colon is now an
      obsolete operation because of the metabolic
      complication and infection. Similar complications may
      occur with an ileal conduit but are less common.

2. a. **Potassium bicarbonate**
      To correct the deficiencies. Requirements usually
      average 2–3g per day and dosage is controlled by
      regular electrolyte estimations.
   b. **Antibiotics** — where there is clinical evidence of
      pyelonephritis.

Paper 10

Question 10.1

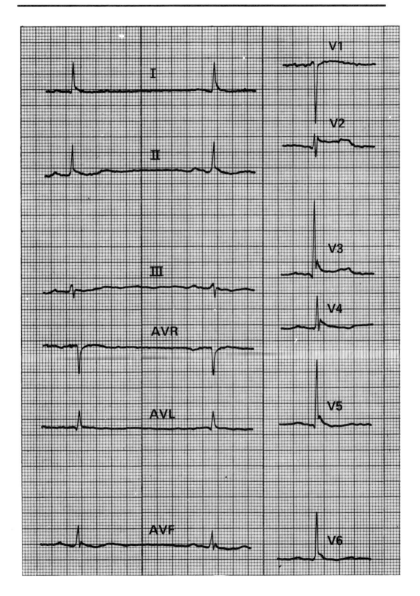

An 80-year-old lady is found unconscious at home.

1. Give five ECG abnormalities.
2. What single diagnosis could explain three of them?

(1) bradycardia   (3) RSR' V₁V₃ RBBB
(2) J waves   (4) T wave ↓ V₄V₅ ANT

Answer to question 10.1

1. a. **Sinus bradycardia rate 32/min**
   b. **Muscle artefact** due to shivering
   c. **J waves.** This is a slurring of the downstroke of the
      QBS complex resembling a reversed J. J waves are
      commonly notched, as seen in V3–V5.
   d. **ST elevation** in V2 and V3.
   e. **Flattening of the T waves**
      The long PR and QT intervals are appropriate for this
      degree of bradycardia.

2. **Hypothermia**
   The first three features are characteristic of hypothermia,
   the J wave being pathognomonic. Myxoedema, which
   can cause bradycardia and flattened T waves, is unlikely
   with normal voltage QRS complexes in the chest leads.
   The second ECG shows reversal of the above changes on
   recovery.

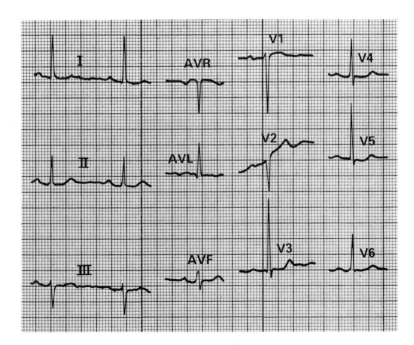

Question 10.2

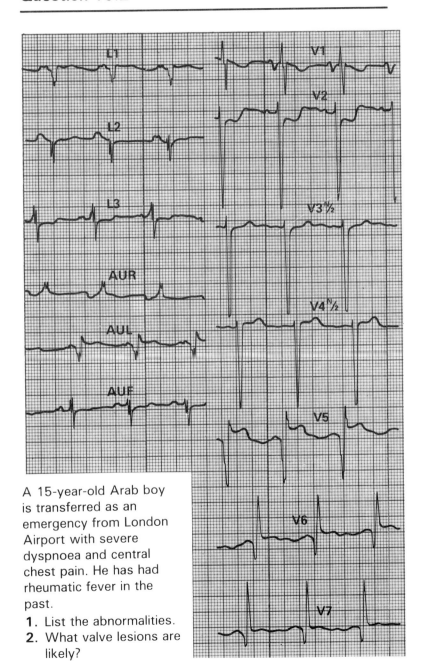

A 15-year-old Arab boy is transferred as an emergency from London Airport with severe dyspnoea and central chest pain. He has had rheumatic fever in the past.

1. List the abnormalities.
2. What valve lesions are likely?

Answer to question 10.2

1. a. **Left atrial hypertrophy**
   There is a prolonged 'M' shaped P wave in lead II and a biphasic P wave in V1. These meet the criteria for left atrial hypertrophy. (See Question 9.2.)
   b. **Left ventrical hypertrophy**
   c. **Right ventrical hypertrophy** is probably also present. He has a tall 'R' wave in V1, strain pattern in the right ventricular leads V1 and V2, deep S waves in leads I, II and III and right axis deviation.
   d. **Q waves and raised ST segments** in I, AVL, V5, V6, and V7 suggesting antero-lateral infarction.
   e. **Incomplete right bundle branch block** demonstrated by RSR pattern in V1.

2. a. **Aortic valve disease**
   A myocardial infarction from any other cause would be unlikely in a 15-year-old boy. The diagnosis is supported by severe left ventricular hypertrophy.
   b. **Mitral valve disease**
   Although left atrial hypertrophy may occur in left ventricular hypertrophy or failure from any cause, changes of this degree, with a history of rheumatic fever, raise the possibility of associated mitral valve disease. Right ventricular hypertrophy provides additional evidence.

Question 10.3

A 24-year-old solicitor is noted to have slight
hepatomegaly and jaundice at a routine medical examination.
Bilirubin 55 µmol/l
AST (SGOT) 19 iu/l
Alkaline phosphatase 56 iu/l
HBsAg   negative
Urine analysis   Bilirubin   +
                  Urobilinogen   Positive
Bromsulphthalein test (BSP):

Time	Serum concentration
15 min	4.0 mg/ml
40 min	1.5 mg/ml
180 min	2.3 mg/ml

1. What is the diagnosis?
2. How may the diagnosis be confirmed?

Answer to question 10.3

1. Dubin-Johnson syndrome

The jaundice is confirmed by a raised bilirubin. Jaundice may be prehepatic, intrahepatic or post hepatic. In prehepatic jaundice (haemolysis) the bilirubin is mainly unconjugated. In post hepatic jaundice the bilirubin is conjugated and there is normally a rise in alkaline phosphatase. The presence of bilirubin in the urine suggests that the elevated plasma bilirubin is conjugated; in this case the normal alkaline phosphatase suggests the lesion is intrahepatic. Normal conjugation of bilirubin excludes Gilbert's disease (unconjugated hyperbilirubinaemia) and a normal transaminase excludes hepatitis.

The BSP test shows a normal fall in serum BSP after 40 minutes but the rise after 180 minutes is abnormal. This biphasic curve is characteristic of Dubin-Johnson syndrome and the second peak is thought to be due to back diffusion of conjugated BSP.

2. Liver biopsy

In Dubin-Johnson syndrome the specimen is greenish-black, with microscopic central zone pigment deposition. In the Rotor syndrome the liver biopsy appears normal. The diagnosis may also be confirmed by measuring a urinary coproporphyrin I: coproporphyrin III ratio >4:1 (normal 1:3) in the presence of normal of near-normal total urinary coproporphyrin levels.

Rotor
synd
|
impaired
hepatic storage
capacity
A R

O-J synd   - Autosomal ? Dominant
defect in biliary excretion mech.   → ∴ no visl^n
of cholan
ogram.
jaundice at any age
pt asympt / vague GI sympt
hepatomegaly

Question 10.4

What single diagnosis could explain these findings?
Calcium 2.8 mmol/l
Phosphate 1.1 mmol/l
Alkaline phosphatase 42 iu/l
Sodium 126 mmol/l
Potassium 5.7 mmol/l
Urea 10.0 mmol/l
Blood glucose 3.4 mmol/l

Addison's

Answer to question 10.4

There are two possibilities:

1. Vomiting with dehydration

In vomiting hyponatraemia is due to salt and water loss with subsequent replacement with water. The hyperkalaemia and uraemia are due to poor renal perfusion secondary to hypotension. The hypoglycaemia is due to starvation and the hypercalcaemia reflects a high total protein.

2. Addison's disease

In Addison's disease, hyponatraemia and hyperkalaemia are due to failure of aldosterone induced sodium/potassium exchange in the distal convoluted tubule. The raised urea reflects the poor renal perfusion and the hypoglycaemia results from glucocorticoid deficiency. Hypercalcaemia is a recognised but ill-understood complication of Addison's disease. It is very rare but responds to treatment with steroids.

Question 10.5

A 36-year-old woman admitted with a DVT. She had a
history of recurrent jaundice and abdominal pain.
Haemoglobin 11.2 g/dl
MCV 103 fl
Reticulocytes 4%
WBC 3.6 × 10⁹/l
    Neutrophils 32%
    Lymphocytes 58%
    Monocytes 3%
    Eosinophils 7%
Platelets 95 × 10⁹/l
Leucocyte alkaline phosphatase score: 12/100 neutrophils
Direct Coombs test: negative
Anti nuclear factor: negative

1. What is the diagnosis?
2. What haematological test is diagnostic?
3. Name one serious haematological complication.

Answer to question 10.5

1. **Paroxysmal nocturnal haemoglobinuria (PNH)**
   There is a mild anaemia, macrocyltosis and reticulocytes
   which in the presence of hyperbilirubinaemia is consistent
   with haemolysis. In addition there is thrombocyltopenia
   and neutropenia suggesting bone marrow depression.
   The negative ANF and Coombs' test excludes many other
   causes of haemolysis. The diagnosis is suggested by the
   associated clinical features of thrombosis and recurrent
   jaundice.

2. **Ham's test (acidified serum lysis test).** In this test the
   red cells are abnormally sensitive to intravascular
   haemolysis, in the presence of acid and complement
   provided from normal serum. There is no lysis in the
   absence of complement.

3. **Marrow aplasia**
   Chronic aplastic anaemia may precede, accompany or
   follow PNH. Occasionally an acute aplastic crisis may be
   precipitated by infections or blood transfusion, though a
   lytic crisis is rather more common. Lytic crises are also
   rarely caused by the administration of iron or alkalis.
   There is an association with myelosclerosis.

Question 10.6

A 41-year-old man with headache. Skull X-ray shows an enlarged pituitary fossa:

75 g oral glucose tolerance test

	Blood glucose (mmol/l)	Growth hormone (mu/l)
0	6.4	28.2
$\frac{1}{2}$ h	10.2	22.8
1 h	11.4	21.6
$1\frac{1}{2}$ h	10.6	24.4
2 h	9.5	24.8

Insulin tolerance test (0.3 unit/kg)

			Cortisol (nmol/l)
0	7.2	28.2	380
$\frac{1}{2}$ h	2.1	30.4	410
45 min	1.8	29.6	405
1 h	2.5	30.8	407
$1\frac{1}{2}$ h	4.6	30.4	395

1. What endocrine abnormalities are present?
2. What other tests should be performed?

Answer to question 10.6

1. The following endocrine abnormalities are present:
   a. Growth hormone excess (acromegaly)
   The resting growth hormone level is elevated and fails
   to suppress (fall to < 2 mu/l) during the glucose
   tolerance test which shows impaired glucose
   tolerance.
   b. Cortisol deficiency
   The cortisol fails to rise above 570 nmol/l during the
   insulin tolerance test, although adequate
   hypoglycaemia (< 2.2 mmol/l) has been obtained with
   a high insulin dose because of insulin resistance. In the
   presence of acromegaly this is likely to result from
   pituitary rather than adrenal dysfunction.

2. The following tests should be performed:
   a. Tests to assess the size of the tumour.
   CT scan: to assess whether the tumour has a
   suprasellar extension.
   b. Tests to assess endocrine function.
   Gonadotrophin levels and testosterone.
   LHRH test if gonadotrophin levels are borderline.
   Prolactin levels
   Thyroxine and TSH levels
   Synacthen stimulation test to confirm that the cortisol
   deficiency is pituitary in origin.

Question 10.7

A 2-month-old child presents with failure to thrive,
hepatomegaly and cataracts:
Urine: positive reaction with Clinitest but negative reaction
with Clinistix
Fasting blood glucose 4.4 mmol/l

1. What is the diagnosis?
2. Give two investigations which would confirm it.
3. What treatment is indicated?

Answer to question 10.7

1. **Galactosaemia**
   Clinitest tablets, based on Benedict's test, detect any reducing substance in the urine whereas Clinistix, containing the enzyme glucose oxidase, are specific for glucose. Reducing substances other than glucose which may occur in the urine include:
   Galactose (galactosaemia)
   Fructose (fructosaemia)
   Glucuronate (drugs or their metabolites which are conjugated with glucuronic acid)
   Lactose (lactosuria)
   Pentoses (pentosuria)
   Homogentisic acid (alkaptonuria)
   Cataracts are found in galactosaemia but not in other diseases listed above. The disease is inherited as an autosomal recessive and is due to a deficiency of galactose-1-phosphate uridyl transferase or more rarely, galactokinase. Other clinical features include: vomiting, diarrhoea, hepatomegaly and ascites, jaundice, mental retardation, hypoglycaemia after weaning and Fanconi syndrome.

2. a. **Paper chromatography on the urine** which may demonstrate the presence of galactose.

   b. **Measurement of erythrocyte galactose-1-phosphate uridyl transferase** which will be low is essential to make the diagnosis.

3. **Elimination of milk and milk products** — the main source of galactose in the diet.

Question 10.8

A 44-year-old man on treatment for a 'kidney complaint' develops postural faints. His blood pressure is 110/60 lying, 70/0 standing. He has pitting oedema of his ankles and sacrum.
Sodium 126 mmol/l
Potassium 4.6 mmol/l
Urea 5.0 mmol/l
Urine: protein + + +

1. Is he sodium depleted or overloaded?
2. What treatment has he been receiving?
3. What treatment would be effective for his oedema and postural hypotension?

Answer to question 10.8

1. Sodium overloaded

The presence of oedema means he is sodium overloaded. Postural hypotension indicates that the intravascular space is volume depleted but oedema reflects an extravascular water and sodium overload equivalent to at least three litres of normal saline. In this case the maldistribution of sodium and water results from hypoproteinaemia due to the nephrotic syndrome.

2. Diuretic therapy

May improve the oedema but does so at the expense of the intravascular volume and may well precipitate hypotension as in this case.

3. Protein replacement

The underlying metabolic defect is a lowered plasma oncotic pressure due to hypoproteinaemia. Treatment should aim to increase serum protein levels by

a. high protein, low salt diet. This is minimally effective but should always be tried as the first step in management.

b. Intravenous salt poor albumin will increase plasma oncotic pressure with restoration of the plasma volume and a brisk diuresis. The effect is short-lived as the albumin is rapidly lost in the urine. It is expensive and should be reserved for patients who do not respond to a high protein, low salt diet and diuretics.

Obviously the renal condition should be treated where possible. However, nephrotic syndrome in adults is rarely steroid responsive.

Question 10.9

An obese 56-year-old male presented with a syncopal
attack associated with sweating:
Haemoglobin 14.0 g/dl
WBC 12 × 10⁹/l
ESR 32 mm/hr
AST 65 iu/l
ALT 18 iu/l
ECG left bundle branch block

Six weeks later his GP refers him with a PUO. His heart
sounds are noted to be soft and he has a left-sided pleural
effusion.
Haemoglobin 10.4 g/dl
WBC 15 × 10⁹/l
ESR 108 mm/h

1. What is the first diagnosis?
2. What is the second illness?

Answer to question 10.9

1. **Myocardial infarction**

   The correct diagnosis is suggested by the raised AST.
   This enzyme can be derived from liver, skeletal muscle,
   red cells or the myocardium. The normal ALT virtually
   excludes a hepatic source and the history, slight
   leucocytosis and moderately raised ESR suggest cardiac
   infarction. In this case the ECG is unhelpful as left bundle
   branch block may obscure anterior infarction.

2. **Post myocardial infarction syndrome**

   3 weeks to 6 months following a myocarcdial infarction a
   syndrome consisting of fever, pericarditis (often with an
   effusion), anaemia and raised ESR may occur. This is
   thought to be due to development of anti-myocardial
   antibodies and results in clinical features indistinguishable
   from the well-described post-cardiotomy syndrome.
   Other features which may occur include pleurisy with
   effusion, pulmonary infiltration and ascites.

Question 10.10

What diagnosis is suggested by the following three Paul Bunnell studies?

	No adsorption	After adsorption in ox red cells	After adsorption with guinea pig kidney
1.	+	−	+
2.	+	+	−
3.	+	−	−

+ = agglutination of sheep red cells
− = no agglutination of sheep red cells

Answer to question 10.10

Agglutination of sheep red cells by human serum is the result of combination of heterophile antibody with sheep red cell surface antigens.

There are three kinds which are distinguished by adsorption tests using ox red cells and guinea pig kidney (rich in Forssman antigen).

1. Antibody that is adsorbed by ox red cells but not by guinea pig kidney is characteristic of **infectious mononucleosis**.

2. Antibody that is adsorbed by guinea pig kidney but not by ox red cells occurs in normal individuals and occasionally in malignant lymphoma. This is the **Forssman antibody**.

3. Antibody that is adsorbed by both ox cells and guinea pig kidney occurs in **serum sickness**.